COLLISION OF RACISM,
NHS AND COVID-19
A Historical Perspective

MADHUN FOOLCHAND

COLLISION OF RACISM, NHS AND COVID-19

Authored by Madhun Foolchand

© Madhun Foolchand 2025

Edited by Marcia M Publishing House Editorial Team

Cover illustrator Jerome McCalla

Published by Marcia M Spence of Marcia M Publishing House Ltd.

On behalf of Madhun Foolchand in West Bromwich, West Midlands the UNITED KINGDOM B71.

All rights reserved 2025 Madhun Foolchand

Madhun Foolchand asserts the moral right to be identified as the author of this work. The opinions expressed in this published work are those of the author and do not reflect the opinions of Marcia M Publishing House or its editorial team.

This book is sold subject to the conditions it is not, by way of trade or otherwise, lent, hired out or otherwise circulated in any form of binding or cover other than that in which it is published. No part of this publication may be reproduced, stored in a retrieval system or transmitted in any form or by any means (electronic, mechanical, photocopying, recording or otherwise) without prior written permission from the Author.

ISBN - 978-1-0685905-4-2

A copy of this publication is legally deposited in The British Library.

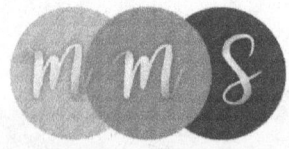

www.marciampublishing.com

*This book is dedicated to my parents,
my wife, children, and grandchildren.*

Acknowledgements

I dedicate this book to my parents. They were born and bred in Mauritius, but their forebears were from Gujarat (India). They were transported by the British to plant sugar cane for Britain and Europe. They were indentured labourers. Others were convicts but a number came voluntarily although their willingness was sometimes obtained by coercion. Neither of my parents talked about their forebears. Both my parents were of working-class background. My dad earned measly wages as a labourer and my mum was a housewife. We, the six siblings, always had a roof over our heads, were always fed, watered, and clothed. I have no idea how my parents did this. On occasions my dad took me to work during the sugar cane harvesting season. I saw him cutting and loading sugar cane on the trucks from morning till late afternoon. This he did for six days a week under the hot sun, rain and cold weather. My dad was locked in the system. The alternative was abject poverty. My mum kept cows, goats, and chicken. My role was to help in the garden, plant, reap and take the vegetables to the local market. That was the only way to survive. Both my parents showed an extraordinary form of resilience. It was my first exposure to the blunt and brutal form of institutional racism. Of course, I did not know it then apart from realising there was something very wrong that was unravelling in front of me.

The other acknowledgements go to my wife, who had to endure my moods during stressful times, and my three children; they supported me in ways that I will never forget. My dear friend Antoine Cyril

Madron and my niece Deborah Hope provided critical comments of my early drafts of my manuscript; their contribution was invaluable. This book is also dedicated for all those who have suffered from COVID-19, especially all NHS staff who died while caring for others. I dedicate this book to all those who experience racism in and out of the NHS and for those who relentlessly fight for social justice.

About this book

The National Health Service (NHS) occupies a special place in the hearts and minds of many British people. It is seen as the envy of the world as it provides care, free at the point of use and is centrally funded. Most of us have been touched in some way from birth, at various times of our lives and even during our last days. Many would have a positive experience while others not so. However, there have been several scandals. The latest being the administration of infected blood to about 30,000 patients. This and other concerns have and continue to receive media attention. By contrast, the existence of racism in the NHS receives scant media attention. Some would react "It's a caring profession, racism can't be there", or "I am a nurse, a doctor and I look after everybody the same" or "we are trained professionals", and among others "we are regulated by our professional bodies". This book discusses how racism was and is alive and well in the country and by implication the NHS. To illustrate this case, I will focus on COVID-19 generally but specifically how Black, Asian, and other minority ethnic people (BAME) patients and NHS staff were significantly impacted.

This book is structured in two parts, pre-and post-COVID-19. The first part discusses the extent to which I experienced racism in the island of Mauritius some 6000 miles away. The existence of racism is placed in a much wider socio-political and historical context. An overview of the presence of Black, Asian, and other minority ethnic (BAME) people in Britain from the 1550s is provided, followed by a discussion of the contribution of BAME people during and after both World Wars. The ideology of white superiority which was developed during the days of slavery featured extensively during the World Wars and percolated into every sphere of British life. As the health service is part of the wider society it is inevitable that all the values and attitudes of white superiority are reflected in the NHS. Some reports have identified inequalities in care provision in relation to old age, gender (women), and lower socio-economic and ethnic minority people. These forms of inequalities have become entrenched in-service delivery. The implication of the fourteen years of austerity fanned the flames of existing inequalities. Other reports have consistently discussed the way BAME staff are and have been treated. When COVID-19 arrived in early 2020, it found inequalities were deep seated and entrenched in the NHS. This was much more evident in care delivery for both BAME patients and staff.

The second part of the book discusses when COVID-19 arrived, it brutally exposed the way BAME patients and staff were treated. Patients and staff were over-represented in morbidity (sickness) and mortality (death) and a disproportionate number of BAME staff died in the course of their duty. This simply confirmed what many had known for decades. The government refused to accept that BAME patients and NHS staff were over-represented in both morbidity and mortality figures. Instead, it published a report to argue that the NHS was a "success story." There is critical discussion on terms 'race,' racism and institutional racism. These are complimented by examples of recent manifestation of racism in the wider society. I propose that this is the most comprehensive evidence of the manifestation of both direct and institutional racism in the NHS. The story is interspersed by my own experience in the NHS as a trainee, qualified nurse, activist, and educationalist.

This book is a valuable resource for health care staff such as nurses, doctors, policymakers, politicians, the wider public and for those who are interested in social justice.

Note from Author

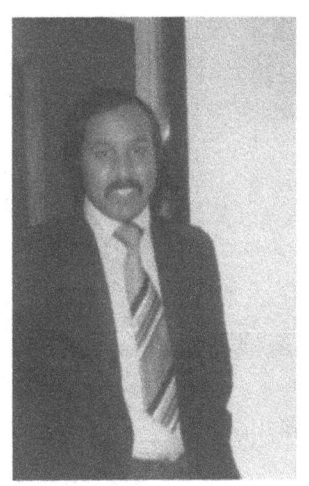

I used various sources to write this book. They include books, newspaper articles, news, TV programs, and websites. I have taken reasonable steps to ensure that these websites were accessible during the drafting period. I am not liable if these websites are later removed.

Contents

Acknowledgements v

About this book vii

Note from Author. xi

Part One: Britain pre-COVID-19 1

Introduction 2

Chapter 1: My early days in Mauritius and my first steps in the NHS 7

Chapter 2: History of racism in the NHS 21

Chapter 3: NHS and BAME patients 47

Chapter 4: An overview of Race Relations post 1948 64

Chapter 5: The contribution and experience of Black Africans, African-Caribbeans and Asians during World War I (1914-1918) and WWII (1939-1945) 85

Chapter 6: An overview of the presence of Black African, African-Caribbean, and Asian people in Britain 106

Chapter 7: Austerity, its impact on institutions and BAME people 120

Part Two: Britain and COVID-19 142

Chapter 8: Britain's state of readiness for COVID-19 143

Chapter 9: COVID-19 and BAME staff in the NHS 155

Chapter 10: COVID-19 and Health Inequalities 175

Chapter 11: CRED Report Fact or Fiction? 200

Chapter 12: Definitions of Race, Racism and manifestations of Racism 231

Chapter 13: Reflection and challenges ahead 259

About the author 271

Bibliography... 272

Part One
BRITAIN PRE-COVID-19

INTRODUCTION

On the 5th of July 1948, one of the most famous institutions was created in Britain. The National Health Service (NHS) was born. Its purpose was to provide healthcare free at the point of use. To this day it is still funded through general taxation, and a smaller proportion from National Insurance contributions. The NHS occupies a special place in the hearts and minds of British people. It is seen as an iconic organisation, and some say it is an envy of the world. Given that context, how can anybody even begin to criticise this much-loved institution? However, behind this shiny veneer lurks a virus called racism. How can anyone start to debate that racism exists in the NHS? The instant reaction would be "the NHS can't be racist, it is led by caring professionals!" or "I am not racist, I am a nurse or doctor," or "I look after everybody the same way," and this book challenges these assumptions and views. The NHS was created to develop a new nation, and this was underpinned by values of being "white". It argues that racism has been present in Britain for centuries and these values have seeped into every institution. This includes the NHS. Racism has been there since the very day the NHS was created and received limited exposure, but COVID-19 brutally and explicitly exposed the manifestations of direct and institutional racism both in the NHS and wider society. This impacted on how Black, Asian, and other ethnic minority (BAME)[1] patients and NHS staff were treated and the rise of hate crime on those who 'looked like Chinese'. This was made worse by the existence of 'hostile environment', the austerity measures and political paralysis when the virus arrived in Britain in January 2020. There has also been a strong body of evidence for decades that the NHS has not provided sensitive and appropriate health care to BAME people.

These were well discussed in the Inequalities in Health (1980), the Chief Medical Report 1992, and the Acheson Report of 2005. The arrival of COVID-19 merely exposed the deep-seated direct and institutionalised racism in the NHS. During 2010-2024 Britain experienced severe economic, austerity, political turbulence and recession. Five factors contributed to these. In 2008 the world economy suffered one of its biggest crises. The Labour government intervened and supported the banking sector by injecting £137 billion of public money in loans and capital to stabilise the financial system. Two years later the Conservative and Liberal Democrat parties formed a coalition government whereby David Cameron became prime minister, with Nick Clegg as his deputy. Both were faced with the dire economic circumstances and needed to act to further stabilise the economy. They implemented one of the most severe forms of economic policies.

---

[1] The acronym BAME refers to 'Black, Asian and minority ethnic' people. It is a controversial term as it groups people from many different religions, cultures, nationalities, lifestyles, views and values. The terminology has evolved over the years, but in the not-too-distant past, terms like 'coloured', "immigrant", "ethnic minority", "Black and ethnic minority" people were used. The latest term is BAME. It excludes aspects like socio-economic background such as social class, age, gender, disability, and LGBTQ elements. It is NOT, by any means, a homogeneous group. Given its limitations and the fact that there is no other term available to date, the term BAME is used in this book, and encapsulates the collective experience of discrimination and racism based mostly but not exclusively on physical characteristics, principally skin colour. This means not being 'white'. The latter is also NOT a homogenous group either as like BAME people, it excludes so many other facets of life experiences.

Severe austerity² measures were introduced. Another factor was an event which was to change the nature of British relationship with the European Union (EU) forever. On the 20th of February 2016, the then prime minister agreed that a referendum would be held, and the British public was to decide if they wanted to stay in the EU or not. The referendum was held on 23rd of June 2016 and 17.4 million people voted to leave the EU. A further factor was the exacerbation of the already existing 'hostile environment.' This was introduced by the Labour administration to "flush out" illegal migrants. Employers were to check the immigration status of those they recruited. The other upheaval came in 2018 when many Black African-Caribbean people who had lived in Britain for six or seven decades were suddenly told they were illegal immigrants. This factor culminated in many people losing their jobs, had their bank accounts closed and among others denied access to services by the NHS. This was and is known as the Windrush Scandal. The next factor was to impact on every British citizen. COVID-19 arrived in January 2020 and found the government asleep at the wheels. As of the 14th December 2023, 233,791 people died from the virus and at least 20,000 died in care homes, very often on their own. BAME patients and staff were over-represented in morbidity and mortality.

Each of these factors individually and collectively impacted significantly on the lives of BAME people in Britain. Finally, 'race' relations suffered a serious onslaught and have been knocked back for decades. Austerity measures have disproportionately impacted on the lives of BAME people, the media, and political activities in the run up to and after the EU Referendum emboldened a vile form of nationalism. They unleashed overt hostility toward both European and BAME people. The Windrush scandal, which was designed and implemented by the

---

² Austerity indicates a policy of sizeable reduction of government deficits and stabilization of government debt achieved by means of spending cuts.

Conservative government, added more fuel into the existing fire of racism and continues to this day.

As a previous clinical nurse, lecturer in health studies, health activist, I invite you to join me on this journey and discover the root causes of deep-seated direct and institutional racism in the country and subsequently the NHS. The claim of racism in the NHS sparks conflicting views. Many would argue that the NHS is a caring institution and therefore cannot be racist. Many who work in the NHS would claim "I look after everybody the same." Others would agree and say "yes, I see and experience it every day." So how does one proceed with this emotionally charged debate? Various researchers could be quoted, and the debate would not be about the findings but about the methodology of how the findings were arrived at. Questions like researcher bias would enter the debate, for example, the sample is small and cannot be generalised, or the method itself is flawed. Many fail to grasp that research itself is not, and cannot be, value-free or culture-free. In this journey I take a unique route. Initially it will involve an exploration from a personal perspective and supported by further research as the narrative evolves. I will illustrate how unbeknown to me at the time, I encountered what is termed institutional racism in my homeland of Mauritius.

This country was formed because of three volcanic eruptions and our journey will elucidate how people arrived there, under what circumstances, and their lived experiences. I witnessed and experienced the last days of the British colonialism in Mauritius. This is complemented by the story of Barbados (previously known as Little England) where my wife, who is the daughter of the Windrush generation, was born. Her parents arrived in Britain during the 1950s. The theme running through these two countries is British history of significant involvement in the slave trade. I illustrate the fact that the ideology of white superiority was developed during slavery days has seeped into every wool of British institutions, and this includes the NHS.

CHAPTER 1
MY EARLY DAYS IN MAURITIUS AND MY FIRST STEPS IN THE NHS

My journey in the NHS started about 6,000 miles away in a small island of Mauritius. It is in the Indian Ocean and was created because of three volcanic eruptions some 10 million years ago. Its size is around 790 square miles and is situated 1130 kilometres east of Madagascar off the south-eastern coast of Africa. It is one of the world's most populated and very culturally diverse countries. So how and when did such a small island get populated? Addison and Hazareesingh (1984) (1) explained that around 1000 AD, the powerful Arab traders were active in the region but there is no evidence they entered the island. The Dutch were the first to attempt to settle in Mauritius in the seventeenth century and their contribution to the history of Mauritius was minimal apart from giving it the name Maurice. They introduced sugar, exterminated the Dodo[3] and stripped the island of ebony (trees) in 1710. The French East India Company laid claim to Mauritius in 1715, renaming it Île de France and began to expand the sugar trade. To grow sugar, slaves were brought from East and West Africa and from Madagascar. They introduced administrative changes, reconstruction, built a harbour and established law and education. The sugar industry thrived under the

---

[3] Dodos once lived on an island of Mauritius in the Indian Ocean. They became extinct less than 200 years after humans arrived on the island. The dodo was bigger than a turkey and weighed about 23 kilograms. It had blue-grey feathers, a large head and beak, and small, useless wings.

French; however, in 1810 the British defeated the French after the seven-year Napoleonic War. Britain's main objective was to protect the main sea route from England to British India. Addison and Hazareesingh noted that most of the units in the armed force came from Indian troops but under British command. After the British conquered Mauritius, the French were guaranteed to keep their possessions, property, lifestyle, language, laws, religion, and customs. As a result, most if not all Mauritians have French as their first language. In 1822, the inhabitants started to be anglicised through the English Language and this language started to dominate the way of life. Nonetheless, the French language remains. In 1807 the British Parliament passed an Act for the Abolition of the Slave Trade across the British Empire. This did not impact in Mauritius. It was estimated that well over 20,000 slaves were brought into the island as soon as it became a British possession. Tharoor, (2017) (2) agreed and indicated that in 1825 the first massive migration of Indian workers from Madras (India) arrived. This was followed in 1835 by 19,000 indentured labourers also from India and continued until 1922. The sugar plantation of Mauritius relied on slavery and its abolition led to a huge demand of workers. The British resorted to India and over the century up to 500,000 were shipped to Mauritius under the contract system. Many were convicts and others came 'voluntarily' though their willingness was sometimes obtained by coercion. My forebears were part of that group. They came from the province of Gujarat. This part of my history is very vague and none of my parents talked about it. My father was an only child, and we knew almost nothing about his parents. My mum has two brothers, and we only knew our grandmother.

My early days in Mauritius and experiencing institutional racism

My father was a labourer and my mum a housewife. I was the third born and had five siblings of four sisters and a brother. We were poor but my parents somehow managed to house, feed, clothe and educate us. My father worked six days a week from morning till evening for measly wages. Sometimes he took me to work with him and I witnessed the sheer exploitation of all these workers. Most were of Indian origin and the pain and exhaustion was visible on their faces. They worked in groups of about ten, under the supervision of other Indian men. The supervisors were the lucky ones. The workers toiled all day in all conditions, planting, cutting, and loading sugar cane trucks. They were exhausted and drained but continued working in the rain and hot sun. How they found the strength to work all day I do not know. It is an experience I will never forget. To make ends meet I worked our land along with my mother. I recall during my early teens that a group of around ten housewives use to meet at a house in the neighbourhood. They developed a system to help each other and used to call it "sitte," in Barbados it is called "meeting!" At the end of the week, their husbands got paid and would hand over some money to their wives. They would meet and pool ten rupees together. This would be a sum of one hundred rupees (our currency) and the women would receive the money in turn; that meant at her turn my mum would get one hundred rupees. This was, at that time, a good deal of cash and my mum would buy school uniforms and on frequent occasions flour. Illiterate and enumerate they may be, but these women were intelligent and found a way of helping each other. This was collectivism in action. This was survival personified.

Mauritius is very culturally diverse. Our neighbours were Christians, Muslims, Madras and other Indian religions. Weekends were mostly taken up with weddings or other religious events. Different languages were spoken all the time and as time went on, we became multilingual. The entire community attended weddings and funerals, and we all knew what to expect. We respected them all. We were economically poor but culturally rich.

Primary education was provided by the state, but secondary school had to be funded privately. I managed to acquire basic School Certificate qualifications. At secondary school we studied mathematics, chemistry, English language, English literature, history, geography, French language, French literature, and religious knowledge. The curriculum was a way of displaying the power of the British and French authorities. We were taught British history and literature along with the French language and literature. We studied novels by Charles Dickens, Shakespeare, the Tudors, and Stuarts, along with the Spanish Armada, and among others War of the Roses. The same for the French literature, books by Moliere were the order of the day. Those were the contents we were to be assessed on to gain any formal qualification. These were not relevant to me. The only subjects with relevance were mathematics and chemistry. I wanted to know more about my own country and how I would survive. It was an instrument used by the British and French authorities to tell us of our inferiority and their superiority. It was an exercise in social control through the curriculum. The latter was an illustration of direct power. We were sold the idea of white superiority. They had a well-designed plan, and it was implemented. The objective was to control our young minds. What made it worse, a couple of the teachers had visited Britain and they frequently told us how wonderful and "civilised" it was. We were not taught of how Indians, Africans, and other people populated Mauritius. In religious studies we were taught the Christian religion. Our religion was of little value, whereas the Christian religion was the "one". In my own mind, I was confused. I wanted to know more about the history of my own family, but somehow, I knew that the Eurocentric form of education was the only way out of poverty.

By contrast the white population were having the time of their lives. They owned most of the land, were at the best beaches, had speed boats, cars, motor bikes, lived in mansions, and had the best jobs in government and banks. The nearest we could get to these places were as cleaners, servants, or porters, every time I walked pass the banks, a feeling of disillusionment would overpower me. I felt lost and helpless. The education for the white people was hugely different to mine. The white schools taught law, land management, accountancy, agriculture, engineering, and other professional qualifications. They had further education in France and/or London. The hierarchy of white superiority was there in our faces, white people at the top and the Indians and others at the bottom. I did not have to read about it, there it was in front of me. The echoes of colonialism were reproduced in employment, in education and in our daily lives. Most shockingly, we did not know it at the time but realised what had been going on many decades later. Equally, there are many of my compatriots who do not or prefer not to realise what happened to them. Many remain influenced by the ideology of white superiority.

Independence and mass migration
There is an old saying that people can only take so much, and they will revolt against any form of oppression and/or injustice. During the mid-1960s, there was groundswell of discontent around the populous and the call for independence began to gain more momentum. India became independent in 1947, Jamaica in 1962, and Barbados 1966; there is no doubt that these emboldened Mauritians to demanded self-rule. After much deliberation, the independence election was held in 1967 and the Labour party won by a clear majority. This led to various ethnic conflicts. Some were reluctant due to fears of domination by the

Hindu (Indian) majority. The strife led to the death of about three hundred people. The conflict was brought under control by the Mauritian army and British forces; the latter were based in Southeast Asia. Mauritius was declared independent on 12 March 1968.

After gaining independence, the country experienced a significant economic downturn. The price of sugar in the international market dropped and resulted in many of the sugar factories closing. Unemployment was rife. Numerous individuals possessing the School Certificate and other advanced qualifications found themselves unemployed. Mass emigration took place between the late 1960s onwards. Recruitment events were held by Australia, and they wanted white people only. France was also an attractive option and was aided by the fact that most Mauritians were well versed in the French language. In addition, recruitment events were held by British health authorities who actively sought applications for trainee nurses to join the NHS. The 'push' factor was high employment in Mauritius and the 'pull' factor was the need for nurses in all parts of the NHS. It later became clear that most were recruited for the Cinderella services of mental health hospitals, learning disability and elderly sectors because these were "hard to recruit" areas. Plane loads of Mauritians left to fill the jobs the British people would not do. On reflection, this was the British plan all along, we were used as a reserve army (more on this later), a term used by Doyal and Pennell (1979) (3). In summary, we have been transported from various parts of India and parts of Africa, initially as slaves then as indentured labourers. My parents toiled for measly wages on sugar cane fields, the younger generation was educated in white superiority, saw all the best jobs occupied by white people, now we were to suffer again. Emigration of so many people can only be seen as brain drain and more importantly by family deracination. Many families experienced separation during this process. I went through the trauma of leaving my parents, sisters, brother, extended family, and friends. When I left my family in late 1971, the family unit was never the same again. On 27th September 1971 I started my nurse training in rural Ayrshire in Scotland. I arrived in a country I knew much about through studying history and English literature but most people in Ayrshire knew nothing about me or my country. When informed that I was from Mauritius, I used to get this blank look and followed by a question,

"Is it near India?"

Another Mauritian man was of African ancestry, and this confused some Scottish people. They stated,

"He doesn't look like you!"

As time went on, we began to challenge these assumptions. We asked,

"How come you are blonde; the other is dark and have red hair?"

Others got more confused when we (the Mauritians) used to talk about British literature and history.

"How did you know all that?"

There was a general feeling that we were seen as less educated.

Baptism of fire in the NHS

I was amid Scottish people all talking in very strange accents. The class was made up of about twenty students, five men from overseas, three Mauritians, one from Nigeria, the other from Rhodesia (now Zimbabwe) the rest were Scottish women. It soon became obvious that the course I was undertaking was a two-year programme which was the Enrolled Nurse (E/N) training, also referred to as the bedside nurse. The qualification was not recognised outside Britain and had no promotion prospects. None of these were made explicit during the recruitment events in Mauritius. The same applied to those who were recruited from other former British colonies and once trained as an E/N nurse, the majority were allocated to the Cinderella services and more likely to be allocated on night duty. The plan was well laid out and we were already doubly disadvantaged, including myself who had more than the required qualification to undertake the three year internationally recognised course. Therefore, I made a formal request to change. The Director of Nurse Education replied,

"Your qualifications are not the same standard as the Scottish qualification".

The fact that we were subject to a very British education was of no consequence. It was not clear how she came to this conclusion but there was no shifting her view. This was an explicit manifestation of white superiority. The Director of Nurse Education refused to accept my qualifications were on par with the Scottish ones. She abused her power and authority to make a decision that was not based on any evidence. This was a manifestation of institutional racism. I was stuck and had to complete the two-year programme of study.

On an elderly care ward, a male patient used to regularly call all black and overseas nurses,

"Black bastards"

He said this with much force, venom, and vile hatred. His face was full of anger, agitation, and overt hostility and on frequent occasions lashed out. How did the elderly man in deep Ayrshire where there were very few if any BAME people know that it was ok to call us racist names. There was no doubt he meant what he said and to whom. This made me feel very angry, anxious and most of all powerless. Where and who do I go to complain about this? There was nothing I could do. I simply had to endure this abuse daily. I actively made every effort to avoid any contact with him and the other nurses knew it. The white nurses would say

"He is a patient". "He is not well". "He does not mean it".

All these implied that I simply had to take the abuse and do nothing. My feelings were irrelevant. They colluded with him. Not one of the white nurses, or ward sister asked me how I felt or told the patient that this was not acceptable. They were bystanders who implicitly supported him. Most laughed, grinned, smirked and thought it was funny. I could not help feeling that some of the white staff enjoyed listening to this patient racially abusing me. For other nurses he used to break out into songs.

There were other comments that I frequently heard. A few catering staff, cleaners and porters would discuss the arrival of "coloured boys" (referring to us overseas male students) very often within earshot of me (and others). It was as if we were invisible yet present. The conversation would evolve in this manner:

"I don't know what these coloured boys are doing here, we have our own boys. Hope our girls keep away from them".

On other occasions we would be warned by people in the village to

"Keep away from our girls".

They must have fallen to the age-old stereotypes about us Black and Asian men. They were not to know that the girls were the last thing we had in our minds. I was amid working where I had landed, or had I done the right thing? During the first six months or so, I was experiencing a series of emotions. I was homesick, felt lonely, and isolated. This was my early introduction of what we now term 'hostile environment'. This was to accompany me throughout the NHS and beyond. The warning signs were there. Over and above these stereotypes, there was a distinct view that we were '*inferior*' and not like them. During a conversation at the dining room table in the canteen, I somehow happened to be in a group of Scottish nurses whose conversation was in full flow. They were discussing a Mauritian colleague who was into the final year of his training. Suddenly they turned round at me and said,

"You are all like us. Aren't you!"

This was supposed to make me feel good. These incidents displayed the manifestations of both direct racism (from the elderly patients and other staff) and institutional racism from the Director of Nurse Education. While we were indoctrinated by the ideology of white superiority in Mauritius, the white Scottish people were socialised in the idea that we were inferior.

A few months before the completion of my course, I applied to about twenty schools of nursing to seek State Registered Nurse training (general nursing). I did not have a single offer. I did the same for the Registered Mental Nurse Training and had about ten offers. I was being directed towards another Cinderella service, yet again.

In October 1973, I started my training to become a Registered Mental Health nurse at a psychiatric institution in the outskirts of Glasgow. It was a 600-700 bed hospital that had patients who have been there for decades. Male and female patients were strictly segregated. The nurse's residence was supervised by a racist warden who took pleasure of patrolling the corridors and harassing the Mauritians and other black students. Nearly sixty students came from Mauritius, Sri Lanka, the Philippines, and parts of Africa. By far, most were Mauritians. Medical services were provided by around five consultants (all of whom were white) and all the junior doctors were Asians or Africans. The hospital was drab, had an institutional feel, and very depressing. The Royal

Infirmary about ten miles away, was a District General Hospital with a better environment, consisted of an Accident and Emergency department, medical, surgical wards and other specialities. It has a teaching and academic department and was a prestigious hospital. I spent almost three months there and noticed that the staff were exclusive of white ethnicity. The contrast between the two hospitals could not have been starker. At the psychiatric hospital, there was no explicit hostility between the white and overseas students but there was an undercurrent and unspoken tension. Further, there were very few interactions between the two groups. I qualified in March 1976 and left the dreadful place the same day.

In April 1976 I started my qualified nurse experience at a newly built psychiatric unit in the Midlands. There were about eight consultants, two from India, one from Sri Lanka, and the rest were white. As per usual most of the junior doctors were Indians, Middle Eastern, and Africans. Most of the nurses were from Mauritius, West Indies, and Philippines and the highest position they were allowed to achieve was charge nurse, yet the hospital managers were all white. This was the hospital I met my wife. She is from Barbados.

Barbados was once referred to as 'Little England' as it had strong connection and a staunchly British attitude. According to World Book Encyclopaedia (1992) (4), Barbados is an island in the West Indies. The easternmost island lies 402 square kilometres northeast of Venezuela. It was created by the collision of the Atlantic crustal and the Caribbean plates. The current view is that the first settlers were Arawak Indians from South America who were driven out by Carib Indians in the 1500s. The Portuguese came to Barbados en-route to Brazil, and it was at this time Barbados got its name Los Barbados meaning the bearded ones. It was named due to the island's fig trees which have a beard like appearance. However, the Portuguese did not settle. The English invaded in 1625, and the first settlement started in 1627. Several English families participated in conflicts over Barbados. They were allocated land and within a few years the island was deforested to make way for tobacco and cotton plantations. In the 1630s sugar cane was introduced and growing it was reliant on slaves who were transported from parts of Africa between 1636 and 1834. The colony prospered and many English families settled there. Barbados initially joined the West Indies Federation of British Island in the West Indies, but this broke up when Jamaica and Trinidad became independent. Barbados gained its independence in 1966 and currently is on a transition to become a republic.

There are remarkable similarities between Mauritius and Barbados. When I visited in 1990, I thought I was in Mauritius. They have been producing boatloads of sugar, from slaves and later from indentured labourers. Both Mauritius and Barbados had slaves from Africa to work on sugar plantations and were exploited by the British. They were both islands with fertile lands, good weather and beautiful beaches. Both countries are one of the most densely populated in the world and gained their independence in the late 1960s. The difference is the language. Mauritius citizens are bilingual, with French being the main language, and Barbados is English speaking.

My wife is part of the Windrush generation. Initially the family lived in Barbados. Her dad left Barbados and went to North America for a few years to pick oranges. Her mother had a job as a servant with the white settlers but ended up working on sugar cane fields. Her father arrived in Britain via North America in the early 1950s. His wife and children stayed behind. After a few years, her mum arrived in Britain and the four children were left with different family members. Gradually the children arrived and joined their parents in the 1960s. Both her parents responded to the 'mother country's' call to help rebuild Britain after the devastation caused by World War II. That was the pull factor, and the push factor was the serious economic downturn after the war and poor yield from sugar cane. Furthermore, many from Barbados fought with the Allied Forces during that war. Once in Britain, they were not entitled for access to social housing and had to resort to private sector landlords. This was further exacerbated by the overt racism and hostility. The practice of "No blacks, no Irish, no dogs" was alive and active during that era. Back then, my wife's parents were in their early adulthood and schooled in Barbados itself. Her father initially worked in London but later moved to the Midlands and worked in a scrap yard until his retirement. His wife found work as a domestic in the local hospital but was cut short due to ill-health. When my wife arrived here, she was in her teens. She completed primary and some secondary education but had no formal qualifications. As jobs were plentiful during those days she found work at a local factory. This she did for a few years but got fed up with frequent strikes and so accepted a nursing auxiliary post at a local mental health unit. As time went on, she attended evening classes and continued her education. After working as a nursing auxiliary for some years, she pursued training to become a State Enrolled Nurse at a psychiatric institution located on the outskirts of the West Midlands. When the children arrived, my wife spent a number of years on night duty. Eventually she did further training to become a Registered Mental Health Nurse and worked in the same unit as me. She also encountered countless episodes of racism from both patients and staff. There were always the frequent comments made such as,

"Go back where you come from".

"Black bastards".

These resulted in little action from managers. There was only one manager that intervened and supported the BAME staff. While my wife was on the verge of retiring one patient openly said

"She will take all that money and take it to Jamaica".

We experienced many racist incidents from patients and staff. With most staff there was always an unspoken undercurrent. There were frequent negative comments made often behind BAME people's back. One nursing assistant resented taking instructions from my wife and other BAME staff. One senior manager made it explicit; he was of the view that only "local" people should get senior jobs. He meant white people. There was no doubt that forms of racism were already well and alive. The British authorities already planned where, whom, and what post they were recruiting for and designed a training programme for many overseas nurses. The few that entered Registered Nurse training reached the charge nurse post but very few moved into management position. Patients, on the other hand, racially abused us with impunity. One could argue that these episodes could well be isolated unpleasant experiences and do not reflect the entire NHS. These episodes must be placed in the much wider context and its roots lie much deeper.

CHAPTER 2
HISTORY OF RACISM IN THE NHS

This chapter provides an overview of the socio-political and ideological climate within which the NHS was conceived. It argues that addressing health inequalities in any form was never the main objective of the NHS. Doyal and Pennell (1979) (1) outlined the precursor to the creation of the NHS. Britain experienced some marked mobilisation in the nineteenth century. The working classes were getting more organised and formed trade unions. They demanded free education for all, the introduction of old age pension and the provision of a health service. This demand grew stronger when it became apparent that many working-class men failed the physical examination tests which were required for enrolment in the army ahead of WW1 (1914-1918). This gave further impetus for the working classes to demand social reforms. They were supported by a few enlightened sections of the ruling elites. Consequently, during the early twentieth century, a series of measures were introduced to improve the health of this section of the population. They were poverty reduction programmes through investing in health of children from an early age. The 1911 National Health Insurance Act was introduced to appease the workers by providing sick pay and a national service for primary medical care. This laid the seed for the creation of the National Health Service (NHS). Unfortunately, Doyal reported that this initiative had to be postponed till after the First World War due to a period of economic depression. The inter-war period exposed the inadequacy of the provision of the 1911 Act and there were calls for a unified system of free medical care. This demand grew during the second World War and plans were being developed for a national health service. The purpose was to 'fight for a new Britain' which led to the development of the Beveridge Report and the welfare state.

The welfare state's main objective was to fight the five giants (also termed evils) that were developed during the interwar periods. They were to fight squalor, ignorance, want, idleness, and disease. It led to the introduction of some public health measures which led to some improvements in general health. However, the welfare state was not designed to fight any forms of inequality. They were left untouched. The main purpose for the creation of the NHS was to develop a 'new' nation. This meant the new nation would be underpinned by values, attitudes, and customs of white people. More to the point, the 'nation building' implied more than a hint of nationalism. Arguably, these were more suited to the values of the middle classes.

Aneurin Bevan led the creation, and the NHS Act 1946 came into effect on 5th July 1948. Many in the medical profession were not in favour of a 'national' health service as they believed it would interfere with their clinical freedom. They were brought on board after having their 'mouths stuffed with gold'. This meant that senior doctors (mainly consultants) could work in both the private and the state sector. General practitioners (GPs) would function as a separate entity although they would still be part of the NHS. The main purpose of the NHS was to provide care free at the point of use, which is still to this day funded by the state largely by taxpayers and National Insurance contribution. However, its progress has been hampered by the focus on curative rather than preventative medicine (Doyal and Pennell). The preventive public health determinants, according to Ratcliff (2020) (2), were and are poverty reduction, environment improvements such as clean air, clean water, affordable housing, availability of suitable public transport, employment, availability of food, leisure, and eradicating all forms of discrimination. This includes racism. The latter receives little media attention.

Asian and African doctors and colonialism.

There were Indian and African doctors in Britain before the NHS was born. Sanghera, (2021) (3) indicated that an Indian doctor practiced as a surgeon in Glasgow during 1845. An African American doctor practiced as a neurologist in London during 1902. Irish nurses were also recruited from Ireland in the years before the NHS. As regards to racism, Doyal and Pennell (1979) provided a historical perspective. During the colonial days the western system of medical education was introduced in Africa. This was to partly offset the shortages of white medical personnel and partially to create a subordinate but well-trained medical labour force. This was based on a hierarchy of race. Europeans were doctors, Asians were sub-assistant surgeons and Africans were assistant medical officers. In Uganda in 1947, a black doctor was paid only a quarter of the salary of a white doctor and half the salary of a white nurse. Visram (2002) (4) and Snow and Jones (2011) (5) argued that many Asian doctors were recruited by Britain during the 1920s to 1930s. Some came to undergo further training and others settled here. By 1945 there were around 1,000 Asian doctors, 200 in London alone and a few practicing in Wales and Scotland. Most, if not all, were allocated to areas with severe levels of poverty, malnutrition, poor housing, and had patients with disproportionate levels of ill-health. Many were heavily engaged in local politics and health campaigns, and provided voluntary services to the elderly as exampled by Doctor Gulati who was known as the pioneer of 'meals on wheels'. The increased reliance on predominantly Asian doctors was triggered by the implementation of the 1911 National Health Insurance

Act. This was funded by a weekly contribution from male workers. It led to increased medical services and a shortage of doctors; thus, Asian doctors were recruited. Kushnick (1988) (6) posited that before the NHS was established in 1948, local selection committees were formed in 16 British colonies. They included parts of Africa, the Indian Sub-continent, the West Indies, and other islands like Mauritius, Singapore, Malaysia, the Philippines, and parts of the Middle East. The creation of a subordinate workforce had already taken root for use in Britain.

1948 (three years after the end of WWII) signalled a watershed moment in British history. It saw some major events that would leave an indelible mark both on migration and the NHS. The British Nationality Act of 1948 was implemented on the 1st January 1949. It gave people of the British Empire, the new status of Commonwealth citizens the right to enter and settle in Britain (Olusoga, 2016) (7). The NHS was born on 5th July 1948, the same year the Windrush ship with 492 people mainly from Jamaica docked at Tilbury, London. The other development was in India. The latter gained independence from Britain in 1947, but it was heavily marred by violence during the partition. Many Muslims went to Pakistan and East Pakistan (later to become Bangladesh), and Hindus, Sikhs, and some religious groups moved to new states in India. The partition led to about 15 million people being displaced and about a million died or were killed by atrocities between Muslims, Hindus and Sikhs (Dalrymple, 2015) (8).

Furthermore, Snow and Jones (2021) stated large numbers of UK-trained doctors (around 30-50 per cent) emigrated to work mainly in the United States and Canada due to relatively poor pay and conditions in the NHS. This was compounded by a serious miscalculation by medical schools of the number of medical staff required. In India, as a direct result of colonial rule, medical schools were taught in English and were geared towards meeting the requirements of the General

Medical Council[4]. These doctors would be eligible to work in Britain subject to approval. The combination of instability during the aftermath of partition and the training provided proved a fertile and rapid recruitment ground for Indian doctors. There was also a smaller number of doctors from various parts of Africa and an even smaller number from the West Indies. During the 1960s between 30-40 per cent of all junior doctors in the NHS were from these countries (Snow and Jones). However, Ward (1993) (9) pointed out that in 1972 the accreditation was withdrawn, and various means were used to call into question the standards of qualification of overseas Asian and Black doctors. Other tests were introduced later on and there is a strong view that they were designed to limit the numbers of Indian doctors being recruited in the NHS. The availability of these doctors was a quick and effective way to rectify the staffing shortfall in the newly formed NHS. The recruitment of doctors and nurses was championed by the Health Minister, Enoch Powell, and even at that point of severe staffing shortages the authorities had a strategy. Black and Asian doctors were directed and channelled to the less prestigious specialities of geriatrics, and mental and learning disability areas (Doyal and Pennell). Snow and Jones pointed out that in the 1960s Powell was a fierce advocate for immigration control particularly from the New Commonwealth. His 'Rivers of Blood' speech in 1968 bears testimony to this. They argued that it was not due to his sudden attack of love and fascination of Black, Asian, and any other members of the New Commonwealth. The recruitment of doctors and nurses not only provided a plentiful supply of cheap labour, but it also reduced wastage. This was used to undermine the shortage argument and strengthened his hand in pressing for a strong line against existing nurses (the largest group of workers in the NHS) pay claim. His overall goal was to keep control over

---

[4] The professional body which dictates the way doctors are trained and the standards they need to reach before being accepted on to the medical register.

public sector pay. In a similar vein, many skilled people were recruited from the West Indies, parts of Africa, and other British colonies during WWI and especially WWII. They were given jobs that white British people would not do. This practice was, and is still very much, the preferred option by the Department of Health and government of any political persuasion. It is much easier to go to the Philippines, India, or parts of the African continent to recruit nurses and other health professionals because it is quicker and much more cost effective. It saves the British taxpayer billions as they have not contributed to the primary, secondary or tertiary and medical education for these professionals. They have been trained at someone else's expense and arrive ready to function after an induction programme.

The presence of mostly Indian, African, African-Caribbean doctors and nurses may well have caused some consternation both to other NHS staff and patients. It may be the first place and time where some staff and patients in Britain came into direct contact with overseas doctors and nurses (Flyn, 2018) (10). Many doctors came with the intention of receiving further training. However, the training offered varied enormously and the distribution of overseas doctors between hospitals and between specialities would appear to minimise their opportunities. On the other hand, the white British doctors had access and received more training. Other overseas doctors were posted as General Practitioners mostly in areas of high deprivation and with poor health facilities. These were predominantly in single-handed GP practices. BBC News (2003) (11) concurred and pointed that many overseas doctors' dreams were shattered very quickly. They did not get posts in teaching hospitals or top fields but found the only doors opened to them were in the 'Cinderella' and 'hard to fill' specialities. Hiro (1991) (12) referred to a study which established that overseas doctors had to apply more often for posts and took longer to gain promotion than their white colleagues. Many were provided with inadequate training opportunities and were set to remain at the bottom of the heap. Kushnick added that the recruitment of overseas born doctors represented a solution to the labour shortage like that adopted by other sections of the British economy. In these cases, labour from the former colonies or from poorer underdeveloped regions were channelled into the richer and developed countries. Thus, Kushnick presented how the poorer nations were and still are supplying valuable labour to the NHS as well as the wider British institutions. The NHS reaped the benefit of trained personnel and the poorer nations, by contrast the provider countries experienced significant levels of brain drain. This practice continues today. The British taxpayer saves and have been saving billions of pounds in this process. This does not feature in the news media or during local, regional or national elections debates. It is another example of convenient amnesia by the British authorities.

The ideology of white superiority was fully developed during the centuries of slave trade. White superiority was reinforced and sustained by various theories, religious and so-called scientific doctrines. These were used to 'justify' and 'explain' the 'inferiority' of black and other non-white people. These belief systems were transmitted and reflected into social structures of society and thus absorbed by most of the populous. These values and ideology found their way into the health service.

During my early days in the NHS in 1971-6, I witnessed some glaring forms of racism. For example, one white Scottish junior doctor was being supervised by a very experienced senior medic. He was Jewish and was soon to become consultant in general medicine. This junior doctor was resentful at being supervised by his senior. He used to get very agitated, angry, and would frequently argue and challenge instructions. There were no warm greetings, smiles, and the junior doctor was visibly hostile even before any conversation took place. There were no informal communications with his superior and he was very often heard making very disrespectful remarks to the nursing staff about this senior doctor. As soon as the medical discussion was over, both went their separate ways. The junior doctor's interaction with other white medics was much more cordial and relaxed. They shared coffee and the general ambiance was very informal. There were no argument or challenges to any decision being made and on no occasion was any negative comments made. The hostility was only with this Jewish senior medic.

In the early 1970s, I was undertaking my mental health nurse training. In that institution all the consultants were white, and all the junior doctors were Indian or African. The general hospital ten miles away was staffed by exclusively white doctors and nurses. Not much changed in the mid-1970s when I moved to the Midlands. The Psychiatric unit had three consultants, one from India, Pakistan, and Sri Lanka. The other six were white. However, almost 90 per cent of the junior doctors were from overseas, mostly from India, the Middle East, and parts of Africa. There were very frequent occasions when these doctors would experience racist abuse from patients, relatives and from some of their white colleagues. Patients would question their ability both clinically and linguistically. Senior hospital managers were oblivious or chose to ignore these incidents and not one of these doctors reported these racist incidents. Some would rationalise and explain away the abuse by saying the patient is "not well" and they do "not mean" it, thereby colluding with their own dehumanisation. A significant number of these doctors were on temporary work visas and required references to seek other posts. Therefore, in this climate they were not likely to complain about any form of abuse or racist incidents.

The first official alarm about equal opportunities in the NHS was highlighted as early as 1978 by the Department of Health and Social Security. It followed the release of the Race Relations Act in 1976 and stated that members of ethnic minority groups were not enjoying full equal opportunities. Many were concentrated in low paid jobs and status, and although they had the requisite qualifications, were under-represented in supervisory posts (DHSS, 1978) (13). In 1990 the King's Fund and the Department of Health conducted a four- year study and found that little had changed, and only a minority of authorities had formally adopted their own equal opportunities policy. They warned that promoting gender inequality would not in itself promote equal opportunity among black and minority groups (King's Fund, 1990) (14).

BAME doctors' experiences

Coker (2001) (15) edited, and with eleven contributors, published a book that gave a wide-ranging account of BAME doctors' experiences in the NHS. She was prompted into this project after she gate-crashed a meeting of largely white male senior and junior doctors, where explicit and over racist comments were heard. The contributors provided a comprehensive account of their experiences. Their views are summarised: detailed accounts of BAME doctors' experiences before they even entered the profession and related their lived accounts daily. Every single case study illustrated the direct and institutional racism these doctors experienced at every stage of their career. One applicant found it difficult to get into medical schools in London despite sending five applications. He suspected racism was a factor but was not sure if this was the case. The applicant was born, raised and educated in Britain, and believed his ethnicity would not be a factor. Eventually, he got a place in the north of England. During his training he recalled being marginalised and described an informal form of segregation where white students gravitated to each other leaving the other BAME students to form their own group. There were frequent instances he was treated differently compared to other white students. Most white students tended to socialise together and formed relationships with senior doctors. This led to the merging of the social with the professional networks and thus provided the students with a more comfortable and supportive working environment. There were also repeated and open racist remarks by medical educators. During teaching sessions on wards, if BAME students did not provide a satisfactory answer to a particular question, they were deemed as incompetent, whereas the white students in the same situation would be given extra tuition. When he raised the issue of racist abuse from patients, he was told he was being "oversensitive", "it's the patients' generation" or that the patients have rights. Effectively, colleagues colluded with the racist abuse meted out to BAME students. He saw how some BAME patients were being labelled and when he challenged this, his colleagues got very defensive and resentful. Although this was an individual case study his revelation resonated with many other BAME students' experiences.

Coker described how others experienced racial discrimination in medical schools. Almost no medical schools published information on their admission processes, namely, data of the ethnicity of all applicants and how many of the different ethnic groups gained entry in schools; attempts to get information were almost always thwarted. Research evidence, naming and shaming through effective use of league tables and political pressure, ultimately led to the decision for medical schools to release information on admissions by ethnicity. This would make it easier to assess the differential impact of admissions by social class, gender and ethnicity, and provide evidence to review and adjust admission policies. After qualifying, overseas and British Black and Asians doctors continued to face more obstacles. After much suspicion that discrimination was taking place while applying for hospital posts, two doctors decided to assess if racism was at play. They developed six CVs; three had Asian sounding names and three with English sounding names. These CVs had identical qualification, experience and general information. They were sent to the hospitals which were advertising for hospital posts. The results were clear. Those CVs with English sounding names were twice as likely to be shortlisted. Yet this project was stopped due to the accusations of fraud. The medical authorities were more interested in challenging the researchers rather than the findings of their work. Qualified BAME doctors were and are still clustered in service posts with limited or no opportunities to gain promotion. Findings from many surveys have been ignored by the medical schools and the wider NHS. In 1999, doctors of Asian origin represented 18.4 per cent of all hospital doctors. The proportion of BAME consultants is highest in the geriatric sector (30.4 per cent). In Accident and Emergency departments they hold 27 per cent and in general psychiatry 24 per cent of the workforce. Their numbers are lowest in general surgery 14.1 per cent, similarly for obstetrics and gynaecology 18 and 19 per cent, respectively. There is also evidence of an over-representation of overseas doctors in less attractive geographical areas.

Overseas doctors, like their UK and EU counterparts, must apply to be on the General Medical Council's (GMC) medical register. Doctors from overseas (outside of the European Union) have an additional requirement; they must sit the Professional Linguistic Assessment Board (PLAB) test set by the GMC. Most PLAB candidates are unsuccessful as it is not simply a linguistic test but also a tough clinical skills test that all non-EU doctors must pass before they can practice in this country. The impact can be that an English-speaking doctor from India must pass this test whilst another from a non-English part of Europe does not. Interestingly, some years later the same PLAB test was conducted with newly qualified British graduates and out of fifty-one, only two graduates were successful. The next statement encapsulates the views of overseas doctors.

"The struggle to get equivalent training for non-overseas doctors is a very real one. Overseas doctors invariably spend their early years on district general hospitals as teaching hospitals posts are largely unattainable. After passing the relevant college exams, the next hurdle is getting a specialist registrar job without which it is impossible to get surgical training and the elusive Certificate of Completion of Specialist Training. Pick a specialty, then see how many overseas doctors are in specialist registrar posts".

There is evidence that many BAME doctors are occupying what is termed Trust grade posts. These are employed directly by the hospitals and are not part of a training programme. There are also concerns about the allocation to General Practice. Many BAME doctors ended up running practices single handed in the inner cities and with heavy workloads because there are more patients on their lists which attract deprivation payments. They also have poor practice premises and been shunned by the majority of white UK trained doctors. Furthermore, there is greater inequality in the distribution of other primary care professionals such as practice nurses and other practice staff. All these increase pressure on the general practitioner. This is another example of inverse care law which means fewer resources are allocated where it is needed most. Despite providing primary care in these areas, a survey indicated about a quarter of patients preferred to see a white doctor. Most of the scenarios above have a recurring theme of racial harassment across the careers of overseas and British BAME doctors. This can be manifested in many ways and the most common form of harassment by colleagues was verbal abuse, being excluded at work and social activities. Others experienced racist comments being made in their presence or within hearing distance. Furthermore, many have experienced harassment from their line managers which was characterised by denial of additional training and career development. The practice of unfair work allocation and the feeling of being over scrutinised and under-supported were highlighted by most practitioners. Moreover, racial harassment was also encountered from services users and their relatives. This took the form of refusal of care or treatment from minority ethnic staff but when staff reported harassment to their managers, they were labelled as troublemakers and consequently experienced victimisation. Managers overall failed to investigate these complaints.

Doctors noted a distinct lack of suitably qualified and professional interpreters. These must be individuals who have a deep knowledge of services users' languages and interpret them in the wider cultural context. The lack of effective communication is a major inhibitor to the assessment, diagnosis and subsequent treatment. This has been an issue of concern for years and has still to be resolved. There is disturbing evidence that points to delayed and inferior medical care for some BAME groups.

These practices go on regardless of discrimination being outlawed by the Sex Discrimination and Race Relations Acts of 1975 and 1976, respectively. The Race Relations (Amendment Act) 2000 does not appear to have any impact on reducing race discrimination and much of the case studies related by Coker were during the late 1999s to 2000. Has the situation changed since? The Royal College of Physicians, (2020) (16) uncovered that BAME doctors faced years of discrimination when applying for jobs after they had completed their Medical Certificate of Competency training. 98 per cent of white practitioners were shortlisted as opposed to 91 per cent of BAME doctors. 29 per cent of white doctors were appointed in comparison to 12 per cent of

BAME doctors. Batty (2020) (17) said many BAME trainee doctors are experiencing "a climate of fear" while in medical schools, amid failures to address widespread racism. In 2020 the British Medical Association argued medical schools were ill-prepared to deal with racism and this led to BAME students being afraid to speak out. In addition, GMC Defence Barristers in 2019 pointed that BAME and overseas-qualified doctors are more likely than their white counterparts to be referred to the General Medical Council in Fitness to Practice cases. The latter has the authority to suspend or strike a doctor for not adhering to their code of conduct. These involve activities in their professional and personal life.

During my days in various clinical departments, I witnessed many incidents when BAME doctors were overtly discriminated against due to their race. For example, some white patients refused to be examined by BAME doctors as they believed that they were not "good enough" both clinically and linguistically. I only recall one consultant who stood out. He heard one patient abusing an Asian doctor. He came out and told the patient "Under the NHS all doctors are equal. You can see my registrar, or you can go". On many instances many BAME doctors would collude with their own abuse by saying the patient is "upset and do not mean it". They hardly talked about these episodes and never reported these to their superiors. The odds were stacked against them. The majority of BAME doctors were on short term visas and needed references to move on to the next post. Most decided not to talk about the way BAME patients were being treated because it does not "chime well with promotion". There were frequent occasions when I witnessed how nurses would make disparaging remarks about mostly BAME doctors. One nurse made it very clear that "there are too many of them" (BAME doctors) here. Another incident that springs to my mindis a weekend with one of the doctors attached to the ward where I was on duty. She was on the General Practitioner training scheme, and we were chatting then suddenly she said,

"Why are so many Mauritian charge nurses. There is one on every ward about." She continued

"they're all standard charge nurses anyway".

She would not expand on her view as to what this meant, but this implied that we were somehow inferior. She was in a relatively powerful position to make this comment. I wondered how would she provide any sort of care for BAME patients when she became a qualified G.P?

Racism in Nursing

When the NHS was established, local selection committees were formed in 16 British colonies. This encompassed regions such as parts of Africa, the Indian subcontinent, the African-Caribbean, islands such as Mauritius, Southeast Asia, and sections of the Middle East. The recruitment of nurses from the African-Caribbean and above colonies began in the 1950s (Kushnick).

My journey in the NHS started in deep Ayrshire, Scotland. It was a predominantly working-class area with men mostly working the mines. There were some semi-skilled workers employed in railway maintenance with school teachers and local authority workers. Over a few months, I realised that many domestics, porters, and Scottish nurses 'knew' that they were 'better' than us. They would be heard talking and made sure we were within earshot of the dialogue. This could be summarised as follows; *"I don't know what these 'coloured boys' are doing here"* and *"they can't be very clever"*. The reference to *'coloured boys'* is troubling. We were all over twenty-one years old and considered to be not men but *coloured boys*. These terms had colonial overtones. White was the norm, and it did not occur to them that white was also a colour. Throughout my time there I never heard the staff refer to white men as *boys*. That label was reserved to us and the hostility that accompanied these words was written all over their faces. There were very few, if any, black African, Indian, African-Caribbean or Southeastern people in deep Ayrshire until late 1960s, so how did they develop the idea that we were inferior to them, and we were *boys*? There was no doubt that this working-class community had already been inculcated into the values, attitude, and stereotypes by all society's institutions. They had been very well socialised in society's norms and infected by the virus of racism.

The nursing class composed of about twenty Scottish women and five black men. Three were from Mauritius, one from Nigeria and the other from Rhodesia (now Zimbabwe). I was soon to find out that these women had no formal qualifications and with this knowledge the colleague from Rhodesia and I asked the teachers some questions. When I challenged the Director (about being allocated to a two-year course) she told me:

"You people come here with nothing and want everything".

She flew into a rage when I stated I had the required qualification. We were told on several occasions that our qualifications were *inferior* as they were not gained in Britain. I asked the Director of Nurse Education if I could transfer to the three-year course. This was flatly denied. My qualifications were *"inferior to the Scottish ones"*. The nurses, porters and domestics poked fun at us and the Director of Nurse Education generously insulted me by claiming that my qualifications were inferior to the Scottish ones. These were the overt racist practices I experienced. It was blatant and continued throughout the entire training programme.

These experiences have some similarities to what Mary Seacole[5] had to endure in the mid-1820s. I was stuck and had no option but to complete the course that had no currency in my country. However, our 'inferior' qualifications did not stop us outperforming the 'highly educated' Scottish nurses in examinations.

Before the two years were up, I applied to twenty to thirty hospitals for State Registered (General) Nurse training. I did not get a single offer. By contrast, I had dozens of offers to undertake registered mental health training. I then moved to Glasgow where the hospital itself was in the outskirts of the city and had a number of students from Mauritius, Philippines, and Sri Lanka. The place was drab, institutional, and very custodial. We (the overseas students) were treated with contempt. We were 'othered' (not "like us" based on our skin colour not being white) and were treated very differently compared to the white Scottish students. Most of the students were from overseas and so were all the junior medical staff. By contrast, the District General Hospital some miles away was staffed by an overwhelming number of white students and doctors. The objective was twofold. The mental hospital was in the outskirts of the city and so were the overseas nurses and doctors. Therefore, two birds were killed with one stone and that meant both the patients at the mental hospital and the overseas doctors and nurses were out of sight and out of mind. I completed my training and left Glasgow the very day I qualified. I started work in a newly built unit in the Midlands and there the similarities continued. Almost 60-70 per cent of the nurses were from overseas. Many of them were charge nurses (ward leaders). Over the twelve years I was there, all but two nurse managers were of BAME ethnicity. Both were made redundant a few

---

[5] Jamaican born Mary Seacole (1805-1881) was one of the pioneers of nursing during the Crimean War. Bringing years of medical experience and combating racial prejudices, Mary set up her own institution closer to the battlefields of Balaclava and nursed soldiers in the fray, winning their ardent praise and respect as she did so. Her contribution has been whitewashed by historians.

years later. The overwhelming number of managers was white men and women. More shocking was a number of them were very inexperienced. I performed my duties in several in-patient departments and soon realised that I needed to update my knowledge and skills. I undertook a degree in nursing studies which I completed in 1988 and decided to move into nurse education. Two white men blocked this avenue. One was the Director of Nursing services, and the other was the Nurse Education. Both obstructed my path for about a year and during that time appointed two nurse teachers who had little clinical expertise. After a few months I was appointed to a nurse teaching post in another part of the Midlands and to my surprise I found out that the curriculum for nurses (general, mental health and children nursing) was very Eurocentric. The curriculum and the staff were not reflective of the population they served. Most of the nurse teachers and managers were white apart from a few BAME teachers in the, yes you guessed it, mental health department! I went over and above in my role as a teacher and held a series of two days training about "health and race". No support was received from my colleagues. They kept well out of it. I frequently challenged senior managers on the lack of "health and race" content in the curriculum and was met with hostility and resentment. This meant that my career progression stalled. Nurse teachers with less experience than me were promoted to senior education managers. More poignant was that some BAME colleagues kept their heads down and did not make any progress in their career.

Racism reared its head again, this time in a comparable manner to doctors. Nursing students used to return to the school after being on clinical areas and predominantly BAME nurses would discuss how they were treated differently. This has been a recurring theme for decades. Many experienced racism from their colleagues and some clinical staff. BAME students were in the margins of the team and did not get as many learning opportunities compared to their white colleagues. This has been recurring for years, and the school staff were very reluctant to take these issues further for fear of "upsetting our partners". Reputation and keeping in good terms with clinical providers took precedence over the welfare of particularly BAME students. Most were left unsupported. As per the advice from the Head of Nursing Education, teachers were required to undertake research projects. So, I developed a proposal about examining equal opportunities, multicultural and anti-racist education in the nurse curriculum. The managers totally opposed this. They believed that it was not *professional and academically credible* to conduct such research. They blocked my proposal for over a year but finally caved in when they ran out of excuses. By that time, other colleagues were well ahead in their research projects. Despite all my challenges and presenting options to nurse educators to prepare nurses to meet the health needs of the multi-ethnic population, little changed. I felt that I could not be party to the miseducation of nurses and left nurse education in the late 2000s. To this day, nurse education is still steeped in Eurocentricity. It is still taught in a Eurocentric environment and by Eurocentric people. The result is that the curriculum has and is still failing to keep up with the local demographic changes. Burnet et al (2020) (18) captured the situation with an outstanding punch line:

"Students are prepared to deal with gaping wounds, broken and damaged bodies, profound grief, disintegrating mental health and much more. We all diminish our professions and academic community if we maintain that openly discussing racism, white privilege and ways of dismantling structural, individual, ideological racism are "too confronting".

This statement encapsulates my experience. More institutional discrimination was to follow. These were among other developments in the Grading and Banding of Nurses, Midwives and Health Visitors.

Nurse Grading and Racism
During the late 1980s there were increasing discontent and frustration among nurse's about pay and working conditions. Many were actively considering taking industrial action. To this end the DHSS (1988) (19) implemented the Grading system for nurses, midwives and health visitors that was designed to provide a career structure and progression. It created a grading structure from grade A to I. The lowest grade (A) would have the lowest skill base with the highest (I) having the most complex knowledge and skills. These skills were to be rewarded with higher pay. Health Authorities were given all the advice and authority to manage the implementation of the Grading structure, and it was to be implemented in 1989. O'Dowd (2008) (20) instanced it worked on the basic idea that pay should be dictated by tasks performed rather than rigid job titles. He continued that the system was not properly funded and there was no agreement between staff and management on the criteria for different levels of seniority. Its implementation was problematic. It resulted in tens of thousands of nurses appealing that they had been wrongly graded. Trade Unions officers worked full time to appeal against the grade allocated and it took until 2003 for cases to be resolved. During the implementation I saw many of my colleagues who were experienced charge nurses being afforded grades which did not fit their skills or sphere of responsibility or tasks. Many were given protected pay for two years while others either retired early, left the NHS altogether, or moved into the private sector. Several of the BAME charge nurses were, over a period of years, moved on by early retirement or resignations and their posts were taken by mostly inexperienced white nurses. Many of those who took these posts were trained by the same charge nurses they replaced. Several of my colleagues complained bitterly about this form of overt and institutional racism. This evolved in front of my eyes and I saw it recurring for years. It was relentless. No one in positions of authority appeared or wanted to see this gross injustice that engulfed the majority of BAME nurses.

Shades of discrimination that Mary Seacole experienced resurfaced in the late 1980s. These nurses were marginalised and discriminated against and were the very nurses who helped various hospitals improve and achieve success. This experience is worth more than any research project. It evolved in and around me. Many of my colleagues suffered and the sense of powerlessness was palpable. Essentially, mostly white managers were given freedom and discretion as to whom they would give the higher grades. I was fortunate because I managed to enter nurse teaching some months before the implementation of the grading structure.

'Agenda for Change' (AFC) was a new system introduced in 2004. It provided a banding structure that applied to nurses and some other NHS staff. It was implemented to correct historic problems with nurses and other staff pay – namely, to provide a more structured way of ensuring NHS staff get equal pay for work of equal value. The banding literally replaced the letters (A-I) with numbers (1-9). The lower bands reflect the level of skills with band 9 being the highest levels of knowledge and skills. Daliwal and McKay (2017) (21) found that BAME nurses and midwives, especially those who registered abroad and recruited by the NHS were underemployed and consequently expressed feelings of loss of self-confidence. This was further compounded by accounts of excessive scrutiny and being under supported. Most BAME nurses lost out on the appropriate banding, and many felt excluded from white networks of power and opportunities for staff development and promotion. They also experienced covert as well as overt racism between the white majority staff and BAME staff as well as 'horizontal racism' between staff of differing ethnicities. The NHS Equality and Diversity Council, (2018) (22) reported minor progress but the proportion of BAME staff in very senior manager (VSM) positions increased from 5.7 per cent in 2017 to 6.9 per cent in 2018. This is still significantly lower than the proportion of BAME staff (19.1 per cent) in NHS trusts. Further still, BAME staff were

1.24 times more likely to enter the formal disciplinary process compared to white staff and in August 2023, GOV.UK (2023) (23), reported similar findings. NHS staff from ethnic minority groups (not including white minorities) were more than twice as likely to experience discrimination than white staff. In 2022, 6.7 per cent of white NHS staff had personally experienced discrimination from colleagues, compared with 16.6 per cent of NHS staff from all other ethnic groups combined. Additionally, 59.1 per cent of white staff in contrast to 49.4 per cent staff from ethnic minority groups thought career progression was fair. So, there has been no demonstrable progress since my days in the early 1970s in deep rural Ayrshire. There are other serious concerns that have had (and are still having) significant adverse impact on particularly BAME nurses and midwives. The Nursing and Midwifery Council (NMC) found some employers referred more men and Black professionals to 'Fitness to Practise' compared to the composition of the register and their own workforce. A large cohort of nurses and midwives felt one or more of their diversity characteristics played a part in the referral from their employer, and a culture of an 'insider versus outsider' left many feeling unsupported (NMC, 2022) (24).

In the latest survey Kline and Warmington (2024) (25) discussed how racially minoritised (BAME) staff face common responses when raising concerns about race equality. Neither managers nor subsequent investigations felt they could state that race discrimination lay behind these behaviours. This resulted in a reluctance or refusal to acknowledge race as an issue. Organisations go to great length to downplay the impact of racist behaviour and there is a lack of empathy. In fact, it is more common nurses are met with frustration, defensiveness and exasperation. Other factors revealed that employers set an unnecessary high criterion for staff to prove any allegation(s) of race discrimination was racially motivated. Tackling race allegations is seen as too difficult, so it is avoided, and equally the process of raising a concern and the time it takes to investigate deters staff from raising a concern. Additionally, there is a lack of confidence in the investigation process that responses will be fair. The survey also concluded that numerous staff lack confidence in trade unions when tackling racism. NHS Confederation (2024) (26) make a financial point. In 2019 the annual cost of bullying, harassment and discrimination was estimated at £2.281 billion, with staff from minoritised backgrounds bearing the brunt.

The NMC does not monitor which bands of nursing staff are referred to the 'Fitness for Practice' investigations. It also has an under-representation of BAME staff at senior levels of the organisation. The NMC Council Members (30 May 2024) had nine who appear to be of white ethnicity and two lay members who appear to be of BAME ethnicity. The Royal College of Midwives (RCM) said their own research showed BAME midwives in London are more likely to face disciplinary proceedings and receive more severe outcomes. This information may come as shock to many, but the situation has been discussed by most BAME nurses and midwives for decades.

Conclusion
This chapter has argued that despite so many policies, legal imperatives, good intentions and commitment racism is not only alive and well but thriving in the iconic NHS. Policies were planned well before many doctors, nurses, and overseas staff were being recruited and directed towards the Cinderella services. The policies themselves were not racist, but their implementation resulted in BAME nurses and doctors being systematically discriminated against. The implementers of the policies were given all the discretion they needed and with little or no accountability. All the policies to deal with or reduce racism have had very little if any impact in tackling racism in 2021.

There are many reasons for this. Two are outlined. Firstly, the systematic racism was and is rooted in the ideology of white superiority and this was and is still manifested in recruitment, allocation of work, and under-representation in supervisory posts. Very few BAME people hold positions of authority and power. All these are reminiscent of the days of colonialism when black, Asian and other non-white people were seen as the 'other' as well as 'inferior' people. These policies were implemented during the days of slavery and are among other examples during the two World Wars. Secondly, there is still a view that BAME staff are a reserve army, as discussed by Doyal and Pennell. An example would be many BAME employees, especially nurses, were 'got rid' of especially during the grading and banding system. Many were downgraded and replaced by less experienced white staff and BAME doctors were allocated to mental health, learning disabilities, and other Cinderella services. It does not stop here.

BAME staff experience racist abuse from patients, and they do this with impunity. Added to this is the systematic harassment, bullying, frequent refusal of extra training and promotion by managers. In addition, there is an over-representation of BAME staff in disciplinary cases by their professional and regulatory bodies. This illustrates a link between direct racism, such as patients abusing BAME staff and the managers using their institutional power to discriminate against staff members. The colonial ideology has seeped into the very fabric of society and the NHS. Hugman (1991) (27) purported over and above supporting the views that ideas of colonialism are reproduced in contemporary health and welfare work. White people are at the very top and BAME at the bottom of the organisational structure of the NHS. He also suggested that professionalisation of health and social care was and is taking place in a climate of continuing racism. The NHS was based on white middle-class values and nation building. Consequently, nurse training or education is extremely Eurocentric. Furthermore, the teachers and lecturers have little knowledge of the extent to which racism exists in British society. Their teacher training and other post registration courses hardly exposed them to the realities of racism. This is a plan to keep and maintain the status quo on one hand, and on the other become a 'professional'. The label of being 'professional' is seen as well intentioned, value-free, culture-free and not impacted upon by the norms and prejudices of any given society. Most work on a "colour blind" basis. It is believed that once one reached the status of a professional there is no need to address sexism, classism, ageism, homophobia, Islamophobia, and of course racism. Professionalism provides a veneer which hides the vile and persistent racism in the wider society and the NHS. This was brought home to me when I decided to investigate the extent to which the nursing curriculum addressed racism. I was informed that "this was not academically and professionally credible." This is another illustration of how institutional racism works. Professionalism was used as a convenient excuse to delay my research. As a previous nurse, I can reflect of a particular incident. A BAME nurse had been racially abused by a patient for days. Most if not all other staff members heard it, knew of this, and did nothing to stop the abuse or support the nurse. One day the nurse reacted and verbally challenged the abusive patient. The nurse raised her voice and was angry. The colleagues witnessed and heard what was said. The affected nurse was reported to the manager. The latter accused her of "being unprofessional" and intimated that she was too "sensitive". It was stated that the nurse needed to be more "resilient" and most of all uphold the "professional standard" required and that she should not take the abuse "personally". The nurse not only experienced racist abuse but also was accused of breaching the "professional" standards. The insinuation can be surmised as "if the nurse were 'professional' and more 'resilient' there would be no need for managers to be involved" and the status quo would remain intact. The manager's duty of care seemed to have been discarded demonstrating that professional standards are interpreted and judged by very senior managers. The over-whelming majority are white men and women both from NHS institutions and the professional bodies (NHS Workforce, 2022) (28). Professional standards in this case took no account of the nature, frequency, or its ideology of the abuse. In addition, it ignored the nurse's feelings. In the final analysis, managers ignored the racist abuse but not the reaction of the nurse. Many have ignored, and still ignore, racism. Professionalism or professional standards are other means and ways to justify the disciplining of the nurse. Professionalism is another way of achieving the same objectives as racism and these disproportionately impacts on BAME staff. From my own experience, I have concluded that professionalism or being professional is linked to managers power and authority. They often set professional standards for others while neglecting to uphold those standards themselves. There is almost no accountability and/or sanction on their actions. The next major question is how does these inequalities and racism in the workforce impact on patient care?

CHAPTER 3
NHS AND BAME PATIENTS

The previous chapters have laid the landscape within which the NHS was created and the values of white superiority which underpinned it. Racism has been discussed in employment of BAME staff. Given that context, how do these impact on patient delivery? This chapter provides four case studies that expose the manifestation of both direct and institutional racism. They are in mental health, maternity, elderly, and haemoglobinopathies provision.

BAME people have experienced health inequalities for decades. Policies to address these have had limited impact. In 1971 Tudor Hart coined the phrase 'inverse care law", and this meant those who need medical and social care the most are least likely to receive it. Townsend, and Davidson (1982) (1) concluded that those from the lower occupational groups had the poorer health experiences in all stages of life. During the early 1970s, the mortality rates of occupational classes 1 and 2 (professionals and high-income earners) had steadily diminished, while those in classes 4 and 5 (low-skilled and semi-skilled manual workers) changed little or have deteriorated. The report also identified inequalities in relation to age and gender (as in women). It also identified higher rates of illness and death among BAME people from certain medical conditions. The report referred to BAME people as immigrants and recorded higher than average mortality and morbidity. The reliability of the data is subject to challenge as recording of ethnicity or race is inconsistent. To explain these differences the report zoomed on socio-economic factors as causative factors. A decade later a more comprehensive account of BAME health was published whereby the Chief Medical Officer (DOH 1992) (2) provided a detailed analysis on various concerns. The analysis drew on the 1991 Census of Population which for the first time included questions on place of birth and ethnicity. The report discussed many determinants of health. These were lifestyles, diet and nutrition, smoking, alcohol use, disease patterns, immunisation, tuberculosis, various infections and blood disorders that resulted in coronary health disease, stroke, poor mental health, diabetes, cancer, stillbirth and infant mortality. The report also highlighted the lack of routine collection of ethnicity data by the NHS and relied on ad hoc studies to extract information. Studies of GP consultation rates and hospital outpatient attendances have shown differences in admission between individuals from BAME people compared to the white population. DOH recommended an increasing recognition of the need for health services to address the needs of BAME people. Positive steps were needed to eliminate discrimination within the NHS and concluded that there are 'variations' in the pattern of morbidity and mortality of BAME people as well as in the use of health services by these groups. Data on ethnicity should be collected and analysed to make informed and evidence-based decisions to respond to the need of this section of the population. This needed to incorporate all areas from health promotion to bereavement counselling.

Thirteen years after the Townsend and Black report, the Acheson Report (Acheson, 2005) (3) concurred. Obesity was added as another concern. Socio-economic factors were and are significant indicators, and the recurring theme of inadequate and inconsistent data collection of ethnicity of patients by the NHS reared its head again. Although making consistent reference to social determinants of health, most of the literature above do not discuss racism as one of those determinants. I discuss this below and how the NHS since its inception has failed to address the health needs of BAME people. It is beyond the scope of this book to identify all areas where the NHS has repeatedly and systematically fallen short in meeting the health needs of BAME people. As a result, four aspects of health provision are discussed. They are mental health and BAME people, maternal health care, elderly care and haemoglobinopathies.

Mental health and BAME people

Significant concerns have been expressed about the experiences of BAME people in and out of the mental health system for decades. In the initial stages it was led by service users and their carers. In my own experience in the early 1980s several 'new' diagnoses were created specifically for this group. These were "Ganja Psychosis", "Cannabis psychosis", "West Indian Psychosis", and among others "culture shock" and could have been applied to any of my and my wife's brothers, uncles, nephews, and other members of our extended family. These diagnoses meant that specifically BAME people were having significant difficulty in adjusting to life in Britain and this caused mental disorder. It would manifest itself as anxiety, restlessness, and despondency and was accepted that black men had "cultural issues or problems", code for 'limited intelligence' and Asian patients were hard to "get through to". As a mental health nurse for some decades, a clinician, lecturer and a member of the Mental Health Act Commissioner[6], I have had first-hand experience of seeing how many BAME patients have and are still being treated.

An Indian lady in her fifty's (who could have been my mother, sister or aunt) was admitted to my ward in a state of "unresponsiveness". She

---

[6] MHAC was a body that was charged to visit mental and learning disability hospitals, interview detained patients, examine their legal papers and make recommendations to the providers.

did not respond to her name, had her eyes firmly shut, did not eat or drink, or use the toilet. She was found to be "medically fit" by her GP and sent to mental health services. She was given basic physical care and continued to be unresponsive for about a week. The medical team decided to wait for her to "wake up" in her own time. The white consultant was at a loss to make a diagnosis and in the end concluded that this lady was suffering from "culture shock". The "treatment" was to repatriate her to India. At no point were the family involved in any of this decision making. He contacted agencies to start the deportation process but then an objection was raised by social services. They had prior involvement with her and her family. There were some family conflicts and when these occurred, she would react by being "unresponsive". The social services intervention was very timely, and the process was aborted. There are some questions which went through my mind during that time. Having worked in a huge psychiatric institution during the early 1970s where the overwhelming majority of the patients were of white ethnicity and predominantly of working-class background, I have never heard of a diagnosis of "culture shock", "ganja psychosis", "cannabis psychosis" or "Scottish or English psychosis". White people were admitted with all sorts of issues, but their culture or ethnicity was not seen as relevant to formulate a diagnosis. Additionally, there were Polish and Irish patients, but repatriation was not considered a treatment option.

On frequent occasions, I witnessed and intervened particularly when young black African and Caribbean men were admitted. Most, if not all, were labelled as being or likely to be aggressive, have taken drugs, and would need a side room and required to be medicated very quickly. All these assumptions were and are still being made even before the patient arrives on the ward. Nurses and medical staff would be very wary of this new black patient (s) and subtly hostile in their interaction. For example, there were limited attempts to talk to these young men to gain an insight from their perspective. Any questions or requests were viewed with suspicion. Usually, a diagnosis of schizophrenia or severe mental diagnosis was, and continue to be, made and high doses of major tranquilisers are given along with other physical treatments. Many are more likely to be physically restrained than their white counterparts. It is common to hear staff refer to these men in negative terms such as, "they are drug addicts, running from the police, beat up women and are involved in gangs" and the list goes on. If two black patients were just chatting, nurses would assume that they are "up to something" and intervene in a very abrupt manner. This may escalate into an incident and potentially result in a confrontation. No such assumptions are made if two white men are doing the same thing. As a member of the MHAC, other commissioners and I have noticed that many locked, medium secure wards and units are disproportionately populated by BAME men who are legally detained. This meant they had no choice to be there. These findings have been supported by research for at least three decades. The consistent findings are encapsulated by the Care Quality Commission (CQC 2010) (4) and their last report concluded that admission rates remain higher than average among minority ethnic groups, especially among Black and White/Black Mixed groups for whom rates were two or more times higher than average in 2010. The 'Other Black' group continues to have the highest admission rate – six times higher than average. In contrast, admission rates have consistently been lower than average among some Asian and Chinese groups, and above average in the Pakistani and Bangladeshi groups. Legal detention rates remain higher than average among the Black and White/Black Caribbean Mixed groups, and among the Other White group. These are supported by (NHSE 2022) (5) in March 2021, the May 2022 UK Parliament (2022) (6).

Once in hospitals there are other worrying trends. The National Health Service Race and Health Observatory NHSRHO (2022) (7) and National

Institute of Mental Health (NIMHE) (2003 (8) reported there is also evidence of harsher treatment for Black groups admitted to inpatients wards; for instance, more likely to be restrained in the prone position and/or put into a seclusion room. There is an over-emphasis on institutional and coercive models of care. The consistent lack of suitable interpreting services has discouraged individuals from seeking assistance, and the availability of culturally appropriate advocacy services remains limited. Ethnic minority groups experienced clear inequalities in access to Improving Access to Psychological Therapies (IAPT). Overall, they were less likely to refer themselves to IAPT and less likely to be referred by their GPs, compared with their white counterparts. There is evidence that inequality in the receipt of cognitive behavioural therapy (CBT) with ethnic minority people with psychosis occurs. They are less likely to be referred for CBT, and less likely to attend as many sessions as their white counterparts. As a Mental Act Commissioner, I found that many clients were often not informed of their rights under the Mental Health Act or did not understand the implications of their detention.

One study that monitored detentions from 1999 to 2016 found that rises in detentions were associated with the economic recession, legislative changes, and the impact of austerity measures on health and social care. A recent systematic review in (2023) found that most common explanations included increased prevalence of psychosis (severe mental disorder), increased perceived risk of violence, increased police contact, absence or mistrust of general practitioners, and ethnicity disadvantages. Cultural barriers, such as mental health stigma and distrust of services is another explanation as to why some people from minority backgrounds may not engage with services earlier or later.

The government reacted and proposed to reform the Mental Health Act 1983. These include approaches to reduce the disproportionate number of individuals from BAME people being subject to compulsory detention and treatment. The proposal brought a stinging rebuke from many members of the National Service User Network (2021) (9), that represented service users, carers, professionals, and communities and raised the existence of institutional and direct racism in their responses at the public consultations. The government failed to grasp that BAME people face racism daily and these are in access to education, employment, suitable housing, school expulsions, experience police harassment, and other determinants of health. It did not take into consideration that stress brought by racism is a major factor that insidiously affect people's health and subsequently impacts on mental health (Fanon 1991) (10). The anticipated improvement from the legislative reform did not work as it was not anchored in any form of evidence, nor did it take account of how so many policies and directives over the last decades have not improved the experiences of BAME people.

There are also major assumptions made about the police, nursing, medical staff, and Approved Mental Health Professionals (AMHPs are those who make assessment and application for the person to be examined by medical practitioners), that is they are culture or value free. This implies that these professionals have not been infected by stereotypes and views of the wider society and the resistance of providers to implement the Department of Health recommendations of Inside/Outside in 2003. The latter provided detailed plans to address BAME issues. All these had little or no impact on the services provided to these individuals. The Race and Health Observatory ignored the fact that clinical judgement is immune to any form of challenge. The clinician is the sole arbiter of the diagnosis and is in supreme authority to diagnose and determine the subsequent treatment. Unfortunately, mental health service provision is not the only area of grave concern as far as BAME people are concerned. Maternal health care has been recognized as a significant area of concern for many decades.

Maternal Health Care

According to Parsons, MacFarlane and Golding (1993) (11), the House of Commons Health Committee raised the alarm about the care of women from BAME ethnicities and those from low incomes and disabilities as far back as 1992; it noted the lack of appropriate support for BAME women. Parsons et al expanded on the above statement by the House of Commons Health Committee that for twenty years, many women have been critical of maternity care. The problems encountered by BAME women must therefore be set in the wider context, rather than being seen as a minority issue. They asserted that assumptions made about the maternity care of these women are often based on stereotypes rather than on reliable information. This is supported by Katbamna (2000) (12) after conducting in-depth interviews with fifteen Gujarati and the same number of Bangladeshi women in their third trimester of pregnancy, identified significant cultural and linguistic challenges faced by both groups. They were impacted by different models of maternal care and the role of women within the home. Communication and language barriers seriously undermined the quality of care. This was compounded by the negative attitudes and behaviour of midwifery staff that also affected the women's experience of their hospital stay. They experienced racist attitudes and behaviours in obstetric services. These are supported by the Race and Health Observatory in 2022 which stated women's experiences of negative interactions, stereotyping, disrespect, discrimination and cultural insensitivity. Equally, system-level factors as well as the attitudes, knowledge, and behaviours of healthcare staff, contributed to some ethnic minority women feeling 'othered' [7], unwelcome, and poorly cared-for.

The other analysis of maternal deaths, stillbirths and neonatal deaths showed mothers and babies from Black/Black British and Asian/Asian British ethnic groups, and women living in the most deprived areas of the country had poorer outcomes. Data from the latest (MBRRACE-UK, 2021) (13) indicated the number of maternity and associated deaths by ethnicity. The data is pooled over a three-year period because the small number of cases meant that the estimated rates can be associated with a large degree of uncertainty. The associated relative risk of death for women from ethnic groups compared with white women is also provided, along with the confidence intervals associated with these ratios. The results suggest that women of Asian, Black or mixed-race ethnicity have an elevated risk of maternal death is more than four times higher than for white women. Birthrights (2022) (14) placed the services BAME received in a historical context. Throughout modern history, Black and Brown people have been perceived by white societies as being sub-human and black women specifically were subject to forms of abuse in healthcare settings. Some examples are medical experimentation without consent and forced sterilisation. The medical model that exists in maternity care today was built on this patriarchal, white-superiority framework. After interviewing 300 maternity staff, received 244 written responses, 11 focus groups of 50 women, 14 in-depth interviews, and polled 556 white and 513 BAME women, it made the following recommendations. It called for all parts of the Midwifery system to: commit to an anti-racist organisation, decolonise the curriculum and guidance, make black and brown

---

[7] Othering is a process that identifies those that are thought to be different from oneself or the mainstream, and it can reinforce and reproduce positions of domination and subordination. BAME people are seen as other due to the colour of their skin. It is assumed that this section of the community is not part of Britain and are seen as 'inferior.'

women and birthing people decision makers in their care. Assessment of a baby's ability to breathe is still using the visual test of being 'pink all over'. This would not provide an accurate assessment for many BAME babies. The wider maternity system should create a safe, inclusive workforce culture, and dismantle structural barriers to racial equity through national policy changes. Brief reference is made to Northwick Park, Morecambe Bay and the latest is the Telford and Shrewsbury maternity services. In 2006, Northwick Park maternity Hospital in north-west London was severely criticised by a healthcare watchdog. This occurred after ten women died giving birth at the same hospital. The Healthcare Commission blamed system failures, weak leadership and a poor quality of care in nine out of the ten cases (Johnson, 2006) (15). In 2021 Northwick Park was downgraded to 'inadequate' following serious incidents, including bullying allegations and baby deaths. Another series of failings were uncovered in 2015 at Morecambe Bay maternity unit. A report by Dr Kirkup (2015) (16) identified serious concerns in the maternity services provided by University Hospitals of Morecambe Bay NHS Trust. This included the death of mothers and babies. The investigation focussed on the deaths from 2004 to 2013 and concluded that the maternity services were beset by a culture of denial, collusion, and incompetence. After making many recommendations, the same Trust was judged as "inadequate" by the Care Quality Commission in 2021. Following this, another earthquake was to hit maternity services, this time at Shrewsbury and Telford Hospitals NHS Trust. The Ockenden Inquiry (2022) (17) was initially designed to investigate the concerns of 23 families' cases, but it grew to nearly 1,500 families, whose experiences occurred between 2000 and 2019. The broad conclusion among many others was thematic patterns in the quality of care and investigation procedures carried out by the Trust. Opportunities for learning and improving quality of care had been missed. All these investigations made detailed recommendations about the structure and management of services, but did not appear to incorporate aspects of ethnicity and, or the socio-economic status of these women and families. Given the fact, deficiencies in those domains have been cited by the Winterton Report at the House of Commons Health Committee in 1992. It is not possible, therefore, to uncover if these biographical data were collected and the extent to which they had any bearing on the care these women and families received. This can be seen as an opportunity missed to include these elements in the investigation and any subsequent recommendation.

Elderly care of BAME people

It has been well documented that Black and Asian people have been living in Britain since 1550s. SS *Windrush* ship brought more people from British colonies in 1948 to help rebuild this country and more were actively recruited to help the NHS to get on its feet. It is not surprising that if many arrived in early adulthood, it would follow that like all people, this section of the community would also grow old. Further, it would be anticipated that health and social care providers would plan for the needs of this section of the community. As discussed above, there is an over-representation of BAME people in the mental health services. However, the elders of the same group seem to be under-represented in the elderly care sector. There is also a view that this is an under-researched area, and it poses questions as to the reason(s) for this. Was there an expectation that BAME people do not get old or was there an assumption that they would have to fit into the existing system? The ONS survey of 2021 estimated the elderly BAME population of England and Wales to be around 11 per cent.

Blakemore and Boneham (1998) (18) posited that it would be a mistake to assume that BAME elders belong to a homogenous group. Like other groups they are impacted by socio-economic factors, social class, gender and disability. Torkington (1991) (19) referred to some surveys which found scandalous shortfall in services for BAME people. She found paucity of Black and Chinese elders who were receiving home help, day care, and residential care. The tendency from providers when asked to explain this shortfall was to inform the minority communities about the availability of the services. The other explanation was that these communities do not use these services because they have strong kinship support or most Black and Asian elders prefer to return to their countries of origin when old. While the latter may be true in some cases, the needs of BAME elders should be factored in all health and social care provision. These explanations can be interpreted as a form of resistance, justification for taking little action, and are examples of institutional racism. These health and social agencies should be very mindful of the fact that many historical and social factors have determined the economic position of BAME elders in Britain. These include the process of migration, settlement and the struggle against poverty, poor housing, living in deprived areas and with poor amenities. All these and the apparent lack of systematic planning of appropriate and sensitive care, are in themselves a form of resistance and evidence of direct and institutionalised racism. When BAME groups accessed elderly services, nurses reported that they,

"Expect you to do it all; you have to bully them, they are very stubborn," it goes on *"they come with trivial issues it is because they have a low pain threshold" Patel (1993) (20).*

The emphasis is *'them'*. BAME elders are not seen as *'us'* or individuals. When I was a health activist, research was conducted by a local authority in the mid-1990s. They found that many BAME people were living in very poor housing, were isolated, and had a series of health problems. Many were not fluent in the English Language. Others were displaying signs of dementia and reverted to speaking in their first language. The research went on to reinforce that there were very few BAME elders in their care or residential homes. They evaluated the diversity training that was on offer and concluded that it ended up reinforcing existing stereotypes that was, and is still, prevalent in the wider society. Commission on Care (2019) (21) reinforced the fact that Black, Asian and ethnic minority older people tend to be poorer, with lower quality housing and pensions, and in poorer health than their white counterparts. BAME older people face additional disadvantages which older white people in similar economic circumstances do not face. Firstly, particularly if they are Asian, some healthcare professionals may assume they do not need help because their families will look after them. Secondly, social care is complex to navigate at the best of times, but some providers still do not make the effort to explain it to those for who English is not a first language. Thirdly, when an older BAME person accesses social care, sometimes does not meet their needs in the way it might for a white person; they experience racism or culturally inappropriate practices which undermined their dignity. Lane (2020) (22) stated that Black and Asian people with dementia are not receiving the same quality of care as their white counterparts. There are also less likely to get medical treatment for dementia. No improvement is in sight. Indeed, the underfunding of social care during the decade long austerity will without a doubt have detrimental effects on BAME elders.

Haemoglobinopathies

Sickle cell disorders and thalassaemia [8] (haemoglobinopathies) are both inherited disorders of the red blood cell which mainly, but not

---

[8] Thalassaemia is an inherited condition affecting the blood. There are different types, which vary from a mild condition with no symptoms, to a serious or life-threatening condition. For the more severe forms of thalassaemia, modern treatment gives a good outlook, but lifelong monitoring and treatment are needed. Good treatment is important to prevent complications developing. http://patientsinfo>...Healthinfowhat is thalassaemia? Accessed 6/10/2022.

exclusively, affect black and minority ethnic people. Anionwu (1993) (23) argued this disorder provided a useful benchmark to assess the willingness and ability of the NHS to meet the specific needs of black and other ethnic minorities. A very brief overview of haemoglobinopathies is provided:

These disorders are more likely to be transmitted if both parents have the 'traits'. In an individual with sickle cell disease, the red blood cell becomes misshapen and rigid, resembling the shape of a sickle when the haemoglobin is de-oxygenated (releases the oxygen to the organs). This process is called sickling and causes a wide range of clinical complications. Normal red blood cells move freely in the circulation and have a life span of 120 days. De-oxygenated sickled red blood cells can get stuck and cause blockages in capillaries (small blood vessels) and have a shortened life span of approximately 20 to 30 days, sometimes less. These blockages are known as vaso-occlusive episodes and are sometimes described as a painful crisis. A sickle cell crisis can be triggered by sudden changes in body temperature, dehydration, shortage of oxygen, and infection. Sickling can result in, intense pain, severe anaemia, tissue damage, infections, strokes, and in some individuals shortened life expectancy. Sickle cell disease requires specialist consultant haematologist or paediatrician (for children) management. Early diagnosis and screening is vital for sickle cell disease. In England the screening year 2019-2020 found 1 in 2517 babies screened for sickle cell disease were screen positive for significant conditions, and 1 in 78 were carriers. This means there is a high number of people that need these specific services. Thalassaemia are usually recessively inherited genetic conditions which affect the quantity of haemoglobin produced. Sickle cell disease and thalassaemia are specific disorders and need specialist and frequent monitoring and management. If managed well and with consistency, life chances would improve and will undoubtedly lead to less complications during the lifetime of the sufferers (PHE 2018) (24). However, this has been met with institutional resistance. In 1976, quoted by Anionwu, a genetic counselling textbook made this statement, "Sickle-cell anaemia is not of great consequence to us in the context of genetic counselling in the UK. The sickling trait and sickle cell anaemia appear to be confined to peoples of African and Eastern origin".

An overview of patients' experiences is summarised by Anionwu. Referring to previous research, she pointed out that not many of the parents of affected children have heard of the condition before their child was diagnosed. Other parents were given very little information and others claimed that they were fobbed off. In some cases, children who developed swelling in their hands and joints (which is an early sign of sickle cell anaemia) were brought to hospital by their parents only for them to be accused to have caused the swelling. During painful crisis patients' accounts of hospital experiences centred on delays in treatment, inadequate pain relief, and for older patients' accusations of being drug addicts. In the late 1980s a patient made these comments, "they know that I have the disease but they really don't know too much about it. I don't think they are interested as it is not a white man's disease." This point is well supported by the lack of tests. Research had identified the inequitable provision of services for sickle cell disease and thalassaemia in comparison with other conditions. There is national screening for babies for phenylketonuria (a disease that predominantly affects white people) and it occurs in 10-12 babies per every 100,000, compared to sickle cell disease in at least 500 in every 100,000 babies of African-Caribbean origin. There are similarities here with white people developing cystic fibrosis. There is a great deal of interest concerning the need for appropriate information, screening and counselling for these diseases but not as much for sickle cell disease and thalassaemia. Anionwu remarked that the NHS has been slow to respond to the well documented and harrowing experiences of families affected by sickle cell disease and thalassaemia. Most drives and initiatives have come from the voluntary sector around the country.

In its report 'No One's Listening' (Parliament, House of Commons, 2021) (25) concluded, "Sickle cell patients too often receive sub-standard care, with significant variations in care depending on which staff happen to be on duty or which area of the country a patient is in".

While care in specialist haemoglobinopathy services (for both sickle cell and thalassaemia) is felt to be of a good standard, this is far from the case on general wards or when accessing Accident & Emergency (A&E) departments. Care failings have led to patient deaths over decades and 'near misses' are not uncommon. There is routine failure to comply with national care standards or NICE standards around pain relief when patients attend A&E. This sub-standard care has led many patients to fear accessing secondary care, or even outright avoid attending hospitals. As a latest example of failures it referred to a patient who was admitted but died in hospital. The coroner stated, "A patient experiencing a sickle cell crisis who rang 999 from his hospital bed after being denied oxygen would not have died if medical staff had recognised his symptoms and treated him sooner" Thomas (2021) (26).

Conclusion

There have been so many reports that discussed the deep seated and entrenched inequalities that exist in the health care of BAME people. Some specific examples have been discussed. There is a general agreement that BAME people are over-represented and sometimes significantly so in most diseases, both in morbidity and mortality. Acheson in 2005 made two broad recommendations. The first was further development of services which are sensitive to the needs of minority ethnic people, and which promote greater awareness of their health risks, and secondly the needs of minority ethnic groups are specifically considered in needs assessment, resource allocation, health care planning and provision. Acheson and Marmot provide a detailed discussion as to the impact of all social determinants as critical in determining the health status of BAME people. This has been exacerbated by more than a decade long austerity measures and it had disproportionate impact on BAME people's health. There is little evidence to indicate that any of the recommendations have been taken on board. All these are not the fault of a few 'bad apples', these are illustrations of the manifestation of institutional racism. Hugman (1991) (27) explains institutional racism differs from personal racism in that it arises not from conscious act but from the failure of practitioners, managers, and in this case policymakers, to recognise the power structures of the everyday world. These are exercised by white and sometimes black [my addition] people without their awareness. Moreover, they fail to take account of the differential distribution of social power. The use of power can be demonstrated by the policymakers deliberately ignoring the abject failure of the Race Relations Act 1976 and the Equality Act 2000. These inequalities and institutional racism have been centuries in the making. Racism in all its forms not only results in socio-economic political inequalities but has direct impact on the way our bodies respond to being constantly discriminated against. The next chapter discusses how racism was already well established during World War I and II, and the little-known contribution of African, African-Caribbean, and Asian soldiers during both Wars.

CHAPTER 4
AN OVERVIEW OF RACE RELATIONS POST 1948

This chapter provides an overview of the major reference points and key events in race relations after the Second World War. 1948 saw the introduction of the Nationality Act, the introduction of the NHS (as discussed in chapter 2), and the arrival of the Empire Windrush which docked at Tilbury, London. At the same time there were developments in India and the West Indies; both of which would have profound impact in Britain. The events discussed are circumstances that led to the Scarman Report (1981), the Macpherson Report (1999), the surge of Islamophobia (2001), the Windrush Scandal (2017), and the under-researched area of the experiences of the Chinese and those who 'look like' Chinese people. They all illustrate the extent to which direct and institutional racism are alive and well in Britain. The term Black, refers to black Africans, African-Caribbeans, Asians, and Indians is used interchangeably.

After the end of WWII, Australia needed to grow its workforce and for £10 POMS (short for pomegranate and linked to migration) many white Britons were able to set sail to start a new life. For many working-class people, the offer of the drab post war and social class structure of Britain was no match to what was on offer; they left in droves. Between 1947 and 1982 more than 1.5 million people set off for 'down under' to opportunity, sunshine and at first some hardship. Winston Churchill pleaded for these mostly young people to stay but his advice was not heeded. This left a shortfall in the availability of workers in Britain (Marshall, 2021) (1). The arrival of immigrants from Europe, Ireland, and the Commonwealth did not cover the shortfall in the workforce (Hiro, 1991) (2). Another development was the implementation of the Nationality Act in 1948. This granted United Kingdom citizenship to citizens of British colonies and meant that anyone born in the empire were British citizens. Their passports gave them the right to come to Britain and stay for the rest of their lives (Fryer, 1984) (3). Many have argued that successive governments have made changes to the meaning of British citizen and were based on racial lines. Irrespective of the Nationality Act, the Windrush ship carrying about 1027 mostly Jamaican people docked at Tilbury, London. They were skilled people who were ready to work and help the 'mother country' recover from the devastation caused during WWII. This was driven by poverty and a very powerful hurricane that destroyed most of the crops in Jamaica and other islands. Furthermore, many had served in the army and the Royal Air Force during the WWII. Olusoga (2016) (4) offered an insight into the political reactions to those who were arriving by SS *Windrush*. Although seen as a watershed moment in British history, it was viewed as an embarrassment and recriminations in high political circles. They pointed out forcefully that these people were not invited and hoped that the arrival was not going to set a precedent to others. It was seen as an invasion of Britain. Olusoga reported that the then prime minister engaged in discussion to divert the ship to East Africa, where the Windrush passengers could work in farms. This did not happen. Hiro instanced that instead of seeing Windrush as free movement of people, they were seen as a sort of slave transportation engineered by evil agencies in the Caribbean.

The implementation of the Nationality Act 1948 coincided with the independence of India. This resulted in the infamous partition (1947) (which led to the formation of East and West Pakistan) and millions of people being uprooted. Muslims travelled to Pakistan with Sikhs and Hindus to India. The resulting conflict led to a million being killed. Many British Indians decided to make Britain their homes. They wanted to escape the severe problems associated by the partition and life free of famine and floods (Fryer).

Despite many job vacancies and the dire need to employ already available labour, Black and Indian people faced persistent hostility. There was much propaganda by politicians and the press. Black people were seen as 'heathens', practiced cannibalism, were sexually promiscuous, uncivilised and had unpleasant manners (Fryer). Hiro argued there was room at the very bottom. These were the jobs local white people refused to do. Very few Black or Indian people were given supervisory roles as white workers would not obey their instructions and the white workers were well supported by trade unions and employers. By contrast, the Polish Resettlement Act of 1947 permitted Polish and other white Europeans to be given much institutional support in housing and education, whereas Black and Indian people found accommodation very difficult to access. One of the most frequent explanations was that their neighbours would resent this. Local authorities had policies that excluded the new arrivals and required applicants to have stayed in the country between one to ten years to qualify for housing. This was a deliberate plan. Most gravitated towards poor quality housing in the private sector which was in the most deprived areas. There was much political resistance to the presence of West Indians, Africans, and Indians in Britain. Politicians were relentless to the point of obsession in reducing immigration and tightened entry requirements at every opportunity. The 1948 Nationality Act has been under constant attack since its introduction. Fryer noted the racist tail wagged the parliamentary dog. Expediency triumphed over principle. In 1964 Peter Griffiths fought on an openly racist campaign in Smethwick (Birmingham) and won his seat with a sound majority. Enoch Powell in 1968 made his 'Rivers of Blood' speech arguing that blood would be flowing in the streets if immigration is not reversed and advocated repatriation. He argued that in twenty years "the black man will have the whip hand over the white man." His main objective was also to erase British history of colonialism. He was dismissed by the Tory leader but gained much support for his views nationally, particularly from trade unions (Hiro). The relentless, cumulative and institutional racism experienced by the Black and Asian community led to several uprisings in 1948, 1949, 1958, 1981 and subsequent years. Hiro reported a series of fights between white and black people in parts of London and Nottingham in 1949. These were not solely due to unemployment because there were plenty of unfilled vacancies despite the increase in the number of Black, Asian and other minority ethnic people living in and around these areas. It was based purely on racial lines.

Hiro reported that during the weekend of 10-12 April 1981, violence and disorder erupted in the centre of Brixton, London. This level of disorder had never been seen in Britain and had been years in the making. In 1919 the government went out of its way to demonstrate that it preferred white and non-British ex-soldiers to Black and Asian British citizens. There were some uprisings between 1919 and 1948 when Black and Asian service people challenged racist practices. These injustices have been transferred to children of the Black and Asian British citizens. There were antecedents that led to the uprising during the 1980s. An economic downturn in the mid-1970s led to high unemployment levels (about 9 per cent), homelessness, child poverty and crime. Black and Asian people were accused of placing strains on already stretched services and by every indicator fared much worse than their white counterparts in unemployment, over-crowded housing, educational attainment and were victims of crime. In 1978 the Leader of the Opposition of the day, Mrs M. Thatcher stated,

> *"People are afraid of being swamped by people from an alien culture and some may respond in an aggressive and hostile manner".*

A direct attack took place on 18th January 1981. Thirteen black people died in a house fire while celebrating a birthday party. There were conflicting reports as to where the fire started. The families believed that the fire was because of an arson attack, the locals believed that it was a racist attack, while the police argued that the fire started inside the property. Olusoga noted the silence from the political class and a strong sense by black Londoners that the authorities were not interested in the death of these black people. Twenty thousand people marched to the police station asking for a thorough investigation. In April 1981, the police embarked on an operation against street crime, they entered a community that had run out of patience with official indifference, ceaseless harassment and vilification. The police used the 'SUS' law which allowed them to stop and search anyone who they suspected were intent to commit an offence. For two days 120 plain-clothed policemen stopped and searched 943 people and 118 were charged with various offences. This was the spark that led to an uprising over the next few days.

During the weekend of 10-12 April 1981 serious disturbances broke out in Brixton which was seen as the most severe form of civil disorder ever seen in the twentieth-century Britain. In the centre of Brixton a few hundred young people, most but not all of them black, attacked the police on the streets with stones, bricks, iron bars and petrol bombs. It was the first time petrol bombs had been used on the street of mainland Britain. The uprising was at its height on the Saturday evening and for some hours the police could do nothing but contain them. Control was regained when police reinforcements arrived. It left 279 policemen and 45 members of the public injured (an underestimate.) Police cars, other vehicles and twenty-eight buildings were damaged or destroyed by fire. This was accompanied by widespread looting in the shopping centre. The uprising spread to Handsworth in Birmingham, Moss side in Manchester, and Toxteth in Liverpool. These were areas heavily populated with Black and Asian people. The government of the day appointed Lord Scarman (1981) (5) to "inquire urgently into the serious disorder in Brixton on 10-12 April 1981 and to report, with the power to make recommendations".

Two views were forcefully made during the inquiry. The first was the oppressive policing over a period of years, and particularly the harassment of young black people in the streets of Brixton. The other was that the disorders, like so many uprisings in British history were protests against society by people who were deeply frustrated and deprived of opportunities. They saw a violent attack upon the forces of law and order as an opportunity to draw public attention to their grievances. He continued that there was a need to consider not only the police problem specific to the disorders, but the social problems which lay behind the uprising. The policing issues were not difficult to identify. What was different was the policing of a community that was multiracial, deprived inner city area, where unemployment especially among young black people was high. Hope was also low.

Scarman concluded that racial disadvantage was a fact of current British life and was a significant contributor to the Brixton uprisings. He pointed out that racial disadvantage and its nasty associate, racial discrimination had not been eliminated. If these are not addressed, he continued, it will continue to be a potent factor of unrest. As regards to the police, he indicated that the "traditional" police methods will have to change to suit the needs and demands of the changing demography of Brixton and by implication the entire country. The police needed to consult and cooperate with the local community. On a general level, he indicated that there needed to be determined ways of eliminating racial disadvantage and racial prejudice in the wider society. The other significant development occurred when a young black man and his friend were attacked by five white racist youths in an unprovoked racist attack in 1993.

The Macpherson Report 1999

The Institute of Race Relations provided the context to this event. It has documented twenty-four racially motivated murders in Britain since 1991. Controversy still surrounds many of these killings and the inadequacies of subsequent police operations, but the Stephen Lawrence case caught the public eye and gained much media attention. This was probably due to the relentless determination from Mr and Mrs Lawrence in their quest to hold the authorities to account. The case exposed the way in which the Metropolitan Police investigated black victims of crime (Barkham, 1999) (6). On 22nd April 1993, Stephen Lawrence, an 18-year-old black man, was stabbed to death at a bus stop by a group of white youths in an unprovoked racist attack. The police failed to bring successful charges against the five youths, who were widely viewed as the prime suspects of the murder. The police were informed and given the names of those who were key suspects the day after the murder. Support to the Lawrence family came from a very unlikely source. The front page of the Daily Mail on 14th February 1997 carried the headline "Murderers"; it named and provided photographs of five men, who it said killed Stephen Lawrence in 1993. The Mail challenged white men to sue the paper (Barkham, 1999) (7).

The other case during this era was the disappearance of Ricky Reel in 1997. This twenty- year-old man failed to return home after a night out with friends. As this was totally out of character for Ricky, the family went to several police stations to report him missing, only for police officers to crack jokes that Ricky had probably run away in order to avoid an arranged marriage, or he may be gay. Mrs Reel stated,

> *"They were stereotyping me and pointing fingers at my race. They carried out this so-called investigation with racist views in their mind."*

A week later his body was found in the river Thames. The police version of what led to his death differs markedly to that of his parents. The latter believed he was murdered in a racist attack. This was supported by his friends who were with him on the night out. They were also racially attacked (Wikipedia, 2024) (8). The latest development is captured by Freeman-Powell (2023) (9). After a meeting with the Police Commissioner on 11/01/2023 the police agreed to re-examine the case. More worryingly, Independent News in 2014 reported later that both the Lawrence and the Reel family were spied on by the police. Mrs Reel summed up her feeling and said,

> *"Rather than helping us pick up the pieces trying to find what happened to us they were spying on us."*

The police surveillance policy is not a new activity. Scraton (2015) (10) reminded us that this has been a well-established practice since the nineteenth century. It was a way of subverting public disorder to contain and monitor the working classes and Irish communities

As regards to the Lawrence case, it took two police inquiries, a public inquiry, and a great deal of determination by the Lawrence family to prompt the then Home Secretary to launch an inquiry in July 1997. Sir William Macpherson, a retired High Court Judge was the chairperson, advised by Tom Cook, a retired deputy chief constable, Dr John Sentamu, the Bishop for Stepney, and Dr Richard Stone, the chair of the Jewish Council for Racial Equality visited Ealing, Tower Hamlets, Manchester, Bradford, Bristol, and Birmingham. All these places had a history of disproportionate number of stop and search by the police and a rise in right wing activities (Muir, 2009) (11). The Macpherson Report (1999) (12) was published on 24th February and concluded that the Metropolitan Police's murder investigation had been "marred by a combination of professional incompetence, institutional racism and a failure of leadership by senior officers". The inquiry found that institutional racism extended beyond the Metropolitan Police Service (MPS). It affected the MPS and Police Services elsewhere and defined institutional racism as,

> "Institutional Racism is seen as the collective failure of an organisation to provide an appropriate and professional service to people because of their colour, culture or ethnic origin. It can be seen or detected in processes, attitudes and behaviour which amount to discrimination through unwitting prejudice, ignorance, thoughtlessness, and racist stereotyping which disadvantage minority ethnic people" (Macpherson of Cluny, 1999).

The report made seventy wide ranging recommendations, encompassing 'Stop and Search' by the police, recruitment, retention and promotion of black and other minorities in the police force and many other aspects of social reform. It was seen as a 'watershed' moment in race relations in Britain. He went further,

> "Institutional racism in the Police Services should not lead to complacency in other institutions and organisations. Collective failure is apparent in many of them, including the Criminal Justice system. It is incumbent upon every institution to examine their policies and the outcome of their policies and practices to guard against disadvantaging any section of our communities".

However, in July 2021 a report published by Parliament (2021) (13) stated,

> "Fairness in all aspects of policing has still not been met twenty-two years on".

As regards to the murder of Stephen Lawrence, BBC on the 18/6/2024 indicated that the four retired detectives who ran the first investigation should not face criminal charges for their actions in the case. The latest review found there was insufficient evidence for a realistic prospect of conviction.

Inquest (2023) (14) is more critical. In relation to the death of Black people the

> "system of accountability for racism and racial discrimination in death of Black people following police contact is not fit for purpose".

It continued, the police watchdog, inquests and the Crown Prosecution Service have historically failed and continue to fail – to scrutinise the role that racial stereotyping might have played in these deaths. Especial focus was to be placed when excessive force is used. The result is that there is no systemic learning and change and more deaths of Black people occur in similar circumstances. Black people are seven times more likely than White people to die following police restraint. The role of racism in these deaths was not substantially scrutinised and officers were not held accountable, and there is no systemic change or learning.

Two years later, Gilmore and Tufail (2015) (15) described the event that unfolded on the 4th August 2011. Mark Duggan a young black man from Tottenham, North London was shot dead by an officer from the Metropolitan Police service. The killing followed a period of surveillance from officers. Mark Duggan was in a taxi and on exiting he was shot twice and died on the scene. All this took place in broad daylight and in a busy street. The media reported that there was a "shootout" and resulted in the police being shot at and a man being shot dead. Duggan was branded by the populist media and labelled as a "violent gangster". At the coroner's inquest, it stated that Duggan did not have a gun in his hand at the time he was shot. Nonetheless, the jury's verdict was that Duggan had been "lawfully killed". The death of Mark Duggan is one of a series of high-profile cases involving the police. Dodd (2021) (16) reported that Mike Cunningham, who retired recently as chief executive of the College of Policing which sets standards for law enforcement said stop and search was the "totemic" issue. He called for "humility" from police leaders faced with sustained criticism after a tumultuous year. He said law enforcement had achieved a lot but had much more to do.

The Muslim community did not feature much by the events surrounding Brixton, the Macpherson inquiry or the Duggan case. This changed by events in the USA. On September 11th, 2001, 19 people associated with the Islamist extremist group Al Qaeda hijacked four airplanes and carried suicide attacks against several targets in USA. These included the 'Twin Towers'.

Rampant Islamophobia

Islamophobia has been in existence for some decades. Allen (2014) (17) defined it as "unfounded hostility towards Islam and unfair discrimination against Muslims individually or as part of a group". This is manifested by fear and aversion towards all or most Muslims. Islam has often been linked to barbarism and a kind of distasteful exoticism in western academic, political and social discourses. In addition, Islam has for many centuries been interpreted as 'the other', seen as inhumane and evil by the West. Although it is not due to race, it is very similar to the manifestations of racism.

Most Muslims have and are still facing discrimination in employment and other aspects of life for decades (Hiro). For many their experiences were to get exponentially worse after September 11th, 2001. This triggered major US initiatives to combat terrorism (History.com editors, 2010) (18). Spalek (2002) (19) outlined the impact on the Muslim community in Britain after the attacks. British Muslims experienced anxiety relating to September 11 even though they were not directly linked to these or future terrorist attacks. They nonetheless faced the threat of being physically assaulted and verbally abused by members of the public. The aftermath of September 11 has shown that events which take place in the global political arena can have a significant impact on their safety and well-being in Britain. For example, Muslim women were particularly targeted by violence and harassment because the act of veiling is a signifier of Islam. Women had their veils pulled off their heads, been violently attacked and verbally abused. These experiences have had a significant impact upon Muslim women's sense of well-being and the negotiation of their personal safety. Many women changed their everyday behaviour, avoiding places that they had not previously regarded as being dangerous. Men, on the other hand, changed their attire in an attempt not to be seen as Muslims. Koch (2017) (20) referred to Change Institute which argued Muslim children were also bullied at school. More disturbing was that since 9/11, during 2003, anti-terrorism laws resulted in 400 per cent increase in stop and search of Asian ('who looked like Muslims') people by the British police.

London was to suffer an attack on July 7th, 2005, named 7 July or 7/7 attacks. It was coordinated suicide bomb attacks on the London transport system. An explosion tore through three trains on the London Underground, killing 39 people. An hour later 13 people were killed when a bomb detonated on the upper deck of a bus in Tavistock Square. More than 700 people were injured in four attacks. The four bombers, seen as 'ordinary British citizens' in the subsequent investigation, carried out the attacks by using inexpensive readily available materials (Ray, 2024) (21). Within most of the law-abiding Muslim community there was at least two different sets of experiences. On one hand there was a sense of anger, resentment, and open condemnation of the London bombing, and on the other, there was an overwhelming sense of helplessness, powerlessness of being stereotyped and labelled as potential terrorists. Hasan (2015) (22) expanded, on an institutional level British Muslims have been spied on, stopped and searched, stripped of citizenship and subjected to control orders and detention without trial. Many were not found guilty of any crime. In another case, West Midlands police told residents the mix of CCTV and number plate recognition devices (which were installed without discussion with residents) were to help cut anti-social behaviour and vehicle crime. The network in Birmingham, however, was being run by its counter-terrorism unit with the consent of the Home Office and MI5. The £3m scheme, called Project Champion, was intended to monitor Muslims entering and leaving the predominantly Muslim areas of Sparkbrook and Washwood Heath. It was halted in June 2011 after an outcry from residents and civil rights campaigners.

The Windrush scandal

The Joint Council for the Welfare of Immigrants (2024) (23) summarised; the 'Windrush' people are those who arrived in the UK from Caribbean countries between 1948 and 1973. Many took up jobs in the nascent NHS and other sectors affected by Britain's post-war labour shortage. The name Windrush derives from the SS Empire Windrush ship which brought one of the first 'large' group (1027) of Caribbean people to the UK in 1948. As the Caribbean was, at the time, part of the British Commonwealth, those who arrived were British subjects and free to permanently live and work in the UK.

The Windrush scandal began to surface in 2017 after it emerged that hundreds of African-Caribbean British people were wrongly detained, deported and denied legal rights. Many lost their jobs, housing, had their pensions and bank accounts frozen. Gentleman (2020) (24) reported on their experiences. Many were placed in immigration detention, prevented from travelling abroad and threatened with forcible removal. Others were deported to countries they hadn't seen since they were children. As these shocking stories hit the headlines, Caribbean leaders took the issue up with then Prime Minister Theresa May. There was widespread shock and outrage at the fact that so many Black Britons had had their lives devastated by Britain's deeply flawed and discriminatory immigration policy.

Many arrived as children on their parents' passports and the Home Office destroyed thousands of landing cards and other records (Merrick, 2018) (25). Consequently, many lacked the documentation to prove their right to remain in the UK. The Home Office placed the burden of proof on individuals to prove their residency before 1973 and demanded at least one official document from every year they had lived here. Those who were falsely declared as 'illegal immigrants' or 'undocumented migrants' lost access to housing, healthcare, bank accounts and other facilities. This harmful and unjust treatment provoked widespread condemnation of the government's failings. Calls were made for radical reform of the Home Office and the UK's immigration policy. In response to these demands, then Home Secretary announced in May 2018 that it would commission a 'Windrush Lessons Learned Review'. It is very odd that the powers that be would "learn lessons" about a policy that was thought of, planned and implemented with surgical precision by the Home Office and with the approval of the House of Commons.

For those who have been affected by the scandal, justice has still not been served. There is a huge backlog of cases still to be resolved. The Windrush compensation scheme is a failure; it is complex to navigate, there is a lack of free legal advice, claims take months, or in some cases years to process, and compensation offers are insultingly small (Gentleman 2022) (26). The policies that led to this scandal are still in place. The 'Hostile Environment Policy' barred those without the right papers from the safety net that can be relied on. Commonwealth citizens were affected by the government's latest version of the Hostile Environment Policy that was implemented in the 2014 Immigration Act. This policy tasked the NHS, landlords, banks, employers and many others, with enforcing immigration controls; they became internal border guards. It aimed to make the UK unliveable for undocumented migrants and ultimately push them to leave. The Government promised to find the "root causes of the Windrush scandal and learn lessons" from it. Wendy Williams, Her Majesty's Chief Inspector of the Constabulary, was tasked with carrying out an independent review. Lawyers, immigration advisors, local authorities, employers and charities, submitted evidence into what had happened and why. The review was published on 19th March 2020, nearly two years since the scandal hit the headlines and its recommendations were accepted by the then Prime Minister Boris Johnson. It made clear that the Windrush scandal was not an accident, but the inevitable result of policies designed to make life impossible for those without the right papers. This, coupled with decades of immigration legislation explicitly aimed at reducing non-European immigration from the Commonwealth, destroyed the lives of many black and minority ethnic British people.

In September 2020, the Home Office published an action plan, that claimed it would 'deliver for the Windrush generation' and usher in 'people-focused policies' in the department. However, the plan lacked substance, was full of evasive language, and misinterpreted recommendations from Wendy Williams' report. There is still a failure to address the most important issues, like the hostile environment and a clear determination to maintain the status quo. The previous Home Secretary Suella Braverman confirmed in a written ministerial statement on 26th January 2023 that the three pledges would be dropped. These were to run reconciliation events, introduce a migrants' commissioner, and review the remit and role of the independent chief inspector of borders and immigration. Furthermore, the government had only fully implemented eight of Braverman's thirty recommendations, while others were partially met. Williams continued, if her recommendations were not accepted, Britain risked another such scandal. On 24th January 2023 in a meeting with the Windrush Working Group, the Home Secretary reaffirmed her department's commitment to the Windrush generation (GOV.UK 2023) (27). There has been a significant increase in the number of claims that received a final decision during 2023. It stood at 2,097 (Waitman, 2024) (28) and over £80 million paid out in compensation in January 2024 (GOV.UK, (2024) (29). There is a distinct impression that the focus was on the amount paid in compensation and not the actual harm caused to black British citizens as a direct result of the scandal. Gentleman (2023) (30) pointed out that the previous Home Secretary had announced plans to close the Transformation Department Directorate. This is the unit that handles changes meant to prevent a repeat of the scandal and were to close by the end of June 2023. The timing of the announcement of the reneging on these components of the Williams review needs to be noted.

Nagesh (2023) (31) reported that the Windrush victims are still being failed by the compensation scheme. The report referred to Human Rights Watch which stated people should be entitled to legal aid to assist in their compensation application. The process is complex, subject to arbitrary decision-making, and just not accessible. The burden of proof placed on victims is unreasonable. It required them to track down employers and landlords in which many of these do not exist anymore. The Home Office, who are the perpetrators, do not have to prove anything. White (2024) (32) indicated that the government admitted that more than fifty victims have died while waiting for compensation.

Gentleman (2022) (33) referred to the origins of the Windrush scandal. It was a culmination of 30 years of racist immigration legislation designed to reduce the UK's non-white population. This claim was in a leaked government report. The stark conclusion was set out in a Home Office Commissioned paper that officials have repeatedly tried to suppress over the past year. The 52-page analysis by an unnamed historian, which has been seen by The Guardian, described how "the British Empire depended on racist ideology to function" and set out how this affected the laws passed in the post-war period. The conclusion was the origins of the 'deep-rooted racism of the Windrush scandal' lie in the fact that,

> *"During the period 1950-1981, every single piece of immigration or citizenship legislation was designed at least in part to reduce the number of people with black or brown skin who were permitted to live and work in the UK".*

It found that the scandal was caused by a failure to recognise that changes to British immigration law over the past 70 years had a more negative impact on black, Asian, South and East Asian people than on any other racial and ethnic groups (Gentleman). Olusoga goes further. He pointed out that while the Windrush ship was on its way to Britain, there was discussion by the then prime minister to divert the ship to East Africa. Another less well-known aspect of race relations now enters the fray-the experiences of Chinese and those people 'who look' like Chinese.

East Asians and those 'who look' like Chinese?

Before the arrival of COVID-19, Matsuda (2021) (34) referred to the work of Dr Anne Witchard, an expert on British Chinese cultural relations. Anti-East Asians sentiments have their roots in history. Discrimination in the UK started as early as the turn of the twentieth century, when Chinese immigrants started to settle in the Limehouse area of London. In 1901, the first Chinese laundry in the British capital opened but the laundry was immediately stoned by a hostile crowd (see chapter 5). Discrimination and attacks against Southeast Asians remained the norm for decades. It sits uncomfortably with the view of how these communities fare in terms of education and household income, as well as other indicators such as low criminality. The tendency is to see these communities as being model minority, so much so that they are not seen as ethnic minority and are not really discriminated against. However, the reality is very different. The undercurrent of anti-East Asian racism plagued Britain well before the pandemic arrived. The lid has now been blown away and given legitimacy to not only to air, but to act on, derision and hatred by violence (Ng 2021) (35). Chinese and East Asian individuals experienced an increase in verbal and physical incidents when COVID-19 reached the UK.

Early February 2020, Campbell (2020) (36) noted that Chinese and East Asian people reported shocking levels of racism just before the outbreak of the coronavirus. British-born Chinese people were seen as carriers of the virus and how people seem to have put a whole race behind the reason for the outbreak. It exposed underlying prejudices towards Chinese people and those who 'look' like Chinese. These comments were blatant and expressed with impunity. Many were verbally and physically harassed in the streets for wearing face masks. Chinese students were pelted with eggs in unprovoked attacks and there were reports of children experiencing racist incidents in schools and on their way to schools. Morris (2020) (37) argued those who looked like Chinese or East Asians were regularly physically assaulted before the pandemic, but the severity and frequency increased exponentially thereafter. Clements (2021) (38) added a Welsh dimension. A representative from the Chinese in Wales Association said a rise in racist incidents have left her feeling unwelcomed. This is confirmed by the UK police data which suggested a rise in racist incidents aimed at Chinese and East Asian people in the last year. Wintle (2020) (39) suggested that,

"Of all BAME people 70% of Chinese people had experienced someone directing a racial slur at them-the highest percentage of all the ethnicity surveyed".

These episodes of direct racism led Townsend and Iqbal (2020) (40) to refer to a police chief who warned that the far right was and is using coronavirus as an excuse to attack East and Southeast Asians. Disturbing as these incidents were, Clements argued that there are considerable under-reporting of racist assaults or incidents. Many ignore these under the view of not "making a fuss". This is seen as the Chinese "conservative" approach and the worry of "getting into trouble". Parveen (2021) (41) referred to the older generation hesitancy to not talk about racist abuse. It is deeply rooted in cultural beliefs, where there is a sense of shame in discussing it. Furthermore, "there is a façade of this model minority of excelling in education and so you kind of shut your mouth, don't complain and keep going". The younger generation Yip suggested, are taking self-defence classes and are ready to speak up to fight racism. The hostility towards East and South Asians was always simmering under the surface but the arrival of COVID-19 emboldened sections of the community to overtly express their anti-East and South Asian sentiments. The authorities failed to stop the widespread scapegoating of this community and to protect them from racially motivated abuse.

Conclusion

This chapter discussed some of the key reference points in race relations after World War II. There is no doubt that Black, Asian, and minority people continue to suffer disproportionately from direct and institutional racism and have done for decades. Both the Scarman and Macpherson reports explicitly discussed the precursor to these uprisings. Social, economic deprivation, and poor educational provision had disproportionate and detrimental impact on BAME people. The police force was severely criticised by Macpherson and labelled as being institutionally racist. There is ample evidence to suggest that little if any progress has been made in addressing manifestations of racism especially in the Metropolitan Police force. Black and Asian communities are still over-represented in stop and search statistics, and the Muslim community face rampant Islamophobia from the wider community. A number of African-Caribbean people from the Windrush generation were suddenly deemed to be illegal aliens. Many had their pensions, and bank accounts frozen. A number lost their jobs, were made homeless, detained in immigration centres and had NHS treatment withdrawn. One factor is consistent, there has been a determined political agenda in Britain to make life as difficult as possible for Black and Asian people regardless of their immigration status. Recommendations from the Scarman and Macpherson report led to few changes. The Williams Report of the Windrush scandal saw twenty-one of the thirty recommendations had been met or partially met. The then home secretary decided to renege on three key recommendations in January 2023. There are similarities in the way the Scarman, Macpherson, and Williams' recommendations were dealt with by the government of the day. The Cameron government wanted to reduce immigration to the '10,000 of thousands' and further promoted the hostile environment. Further still, a van was driven around parts of London advising "In the UK illegally? Go home or face arrest" and the Home Office destroyed the landing cards of some who arrived by Windrush. During COVID-19 pandemic, members of the Chinese and those who 'look like' Chinese people was targeted. These hostilities have been years in the making. The next chapter discusses the contribution and experiences of Black, Indian, and other minorities during the two World Wars.

CHAPTER 5
THE CONTRIBUTION AND EXPERIENCE OF BLACK AFRICANS, AFRICAN-CARIBBEANS AND ASIANS DURING WORLD WAR I (1914-1918) AND WWII (1939-1945)

This chapter discusses how the values, attitudes, and deeply held views of Asians, Africans and African-Caribbeans formed during slavery and indentured labouring period were reproduced during the World Wars. Wilkinson and Pickett (2010) (1) added another dimension; they postulated that during both World Wars, there were full employment and considerable narrower income differences - the result of deliberate government policies to promote co-operation with the war effort. During World War II, working-class income rose by 9 per cent and the middle class fell by 7 per cent. Rates of relative poverty were halved, while the resulting sense of camaraderie and social cohesion prevailed. None of these percolated into the lives of Black African, African-Caribbean, and Asian people during and after the Wars. Visram (2002) (2) argued that race superiority was well supported by biological based pseudoscience. These deeply held values and attitudes are still significantly impacting on day-to-day lives of the above people and communities.

There was and still is a view in the West that both wars are referred to as a 'White Man's War'. Olusoga (2016) (3) argued the First World War (WWI) started in Africa and ended in Africa. On 12th August 1914, a small British force headed through the African bush towards the capital of a German colony where a soldier from the British West African Frontier Force fired the first shot. WWI began in Africa and in ended there on 14th November 1918. During WWI, black people from Africa, the African-Caribbean countries, and India gained a new and first-hand experience of the racism and racial hierarchies that informed, and for many 'justified', colonial rule. This was in some ways not easily foreseeable as WWI led to a lowering of physical, cultural, and legal barriers that were created before. One million African men were recruited by Britain to work as carriers in Africa. Thousands of men from modern Ghana fought the Germans in East Africa. Other Africans from Sudan, Rhodesia (now Zimbabwe) Ethiopia, and Nyasaland (now Malawi) were recruited to fight the Germans. When these soldiers met, they were able to discuss their experiences and gained a new, deeper understanding of the workings of the empire. This combined with deep resentment at the unequal and unjust treatment black and Asian soldiers and sailors experienced during the War. Consequently, many were very disillusioned and returned to their homes. Olusoga related most African-Caribbeans were actively recruited to join the 'mother country' and fight the German army during WWI. On the domestic level there was much poverty which was a 'push' factor for many African-Caribbeans to join the forces, and many paid their own fares to Britain. Three weeks into the war, the War Office was asked to consider a contingent of troops from African-Caribbean countries be sent to serve abroad. The War Office questioned the fighting ability of these black men and their ability to withstand the cold of a European winter. It was suggested that these men would be better used to maintain order in the islands of the West Indies.

The War Office regarded African-Caribbeans in the British army as highly undesirable and called the Colonial Office to discourage volunteers from believing that if they travelled to Britain they would be welcomed into the army. The only exception was the British Indian army. They emerged out of the Indian Mutiny and occupied a unique place in the Empire. There was a determination in the War Office and white settlers in Africa that black Africans and African-Caribbeans were not to be permitted to fight against white men due to fear; it would undermine white racial prestige and threaten the security of white settlers in the colonies. For decades, the colonial administration made every effort to ensure that modern weapons were kept out of the hands of their black subjects and impressed upon them that white lives were sacrosanct. Black men were armed only when formed into colonial regiments and used to fight other Africans under the watchful eyes of white officers. As the war progressed the numbers of the British West Indian Regiment were raised, coming from most parts of the West Indies with the majority being Jamaicans. Many of these men were rejected on medical grounds. The Brigadier then commented that, "these men only came in for a meal." However, once trained they caught the eye of the press and the public and were soon posted to Egypt as it was presumed that they would be able to withstand the heat better than white British soldiers. In 1916, a couple of battalions were sent to France expecting to fight. They found that they were segregated from the white British troops and became a labour battalion. Most dug, repaired and worked in the munitions depots and faced racist taunts from white troops. Enormous efforts were made to keep these men in their lowly position at the foot of the imagined hierarchy of races. Even when faced with an acute manpower shortage, the British unlike the French put racial considerations above all other factors and refused to recruit black Africans and African-Caribbeans for combat in Europe. The Indians soldiers, on the other hand, were welcomed.

Olusoga asserted even after British casualties began to mount alarmingly, the British still refused to allow the deployment of African and African-Caribbeans soldiers. In contrast, France was very active in recruiting men from parts of Africa and deployed them in Europe to take part in French attacks. The British continued to maintain that "a large body of trained and disciplined black men would create obvious difficulties and might seriously menace the supremacy of the white". They added, "no South African native could stand the European winter", this theme constantly repeated by British politicians and colonial administrators right up until 1940s. This did not stand the test of scrutiny as the European winter did not interfere with the performance of African soldiers in France. The latter proved while fighting for the French that they had been meeting these challenges for some years.

In 1916, the Battle of Somme (which lasted four hundred and forty days) generated casualty lists far longer than anticipated. The volunteers that swelled the ranks in 1915 were decimated. Despite this manpower crisis the War Office and the Chief of Staff were still resistant to recruiting African soldiers. The soldiers themselves were eager to join in the hope that their contribution would lead to the negotiation of a better deal with the post-war empire. There was also a growing view from some quarters that a change of mindset was needed. Others argued there were 100,000 Africans with training who would be ready to fight the Germans, but this did not chime well with what was evolving in mainland Britain. Thousands of British people volunteered for service in 1914 and 1915, but a shocking number were found to be unfit for military purposes. This was reported to be about 60 percent. Furthermore, by the end of 1916, fifty thousand British troops were being treated for shell shock. Even during these desperate times there were still strong resistance for the involvement of African soldiers. It was believed that black African men fighting alongside emaciated white men would challenge the supremacy of the white race and that would be seen as the end of white supremacy. These were the ideology and the stereotypes that those in power were not prepared to challenge. They simply colluded with them. It was not until a British official accepted an invitation and visited the French camps that he was persuaded of the ability of these Africans who were successfully fighting on the frontline. More support was given from various politicians for the recruitment of African soldiers, but they still faced resistance from the army hierarchy. Nonetheless, many found their way into the armed forces by travelling to Britain and successfully enlisted in the British Army Units and the Royal Air Force. This was facilitated by some recruiting officers who were more willing to accept Africans (Olusoga). Others were able to cross the colour line and joined the army were black men already in Britain before the start of the war, and incrementally black recruits could be found in all branches of the armed forces. Edencamp (2021) (4) indicated that 60,000 black South Africans and 120,000 other Africans were in the British army in Africa. This was supplemented by 16,000 African-Caribbeans who donated large sums of money to aid the war effort. Olusoga reminded us of another valuable input made by seamen from all parts of the commonwealth. The merchant shipping that had been Britain's lifeline and the fleet that had enforced the blockade of her enemies had been manned by Chinese seamen from across the empire including Africa and the African-Caribbean countries. These blockades maintain Britain with food supplies, while Germany suffered by 'hunger blockade'.

Despite contributing money and men towards the war, opponents having succeeded in preventing the deployment of black men on the European battlefield, the British authorities continued to ignore the role played by these soldiers. They were determined to airbrush the contribution of these black men towards the war efforts. In the Victory Parade held on the 19th July 1919, Olusoga and Barnett Group related that these black men were excluded. No troops from the African-Caribbean countries or the Black African units were permitted to march. When asked why this occurred, the colonial office stated it would be impolite to bring to England coloured detachments to participate in peace processions. These troops were also excluded from further events. Williams, (2018) (5) added the African American veterans contributed during WWI with the hope that their service would secure their civil rights at home. The British authorities were determined to also deliberately wipe out the contribution of these black men during WWI.

Black African, and African-Caribbean soldiers after the end of WWI

Hiro (1991) (6) challenged an extremely popular myth about the reaction to the presence of black people in Britain. It is commonly argued that white people's hostility towards Black and Asian people is related to the size of that community. As early as 1596, Queen Elizabeth I requested that Lord Mayors of various towns to deport the blackamoores even when there were a few thousand Black or Asian people. Most were brought by the rich and famous and were in the main servants and musicians. The population of Britain at that time was around 3,000,000. Fryer, (1984) (7) argued that when the armistice was signalled on 11th November 1918, the war time boom for black labour fizzled out as quickly as it had begun. Olusoga reported that many black soldiers who returned to Italy from Egypt were ordered to do the laundry both for the white British troops, civilian labourers, and then clean the latrines. Black soldiers were instantly demoted to labourers, denied pay increases, and only received increase in pay after a mutiny, while some were imprisoned, and one was executed by the firing squad.

Hiro stated that this led to the first 'race riot' or uprising which took place in 1919 in Liverpool. The black population at that time was estimated at around 2,000 to 5,000 (Fryer). The uprising quickly spread to all the dock areas where Black and Asian people lived in Cardiff, Manchester, Glasgow, Hull, and London. There were about 30,000 Africans, West Indians, Arabs, Chinese, Filipinos, Greeks, Somalis, and Asians, all non-Europeans in these areas. The rioting consisted of white people attacking the person and the property of black and other non-European people. The terrified victims tried to defend themselves as best they could. More fuel was added to the fire when, according to Olusoga, a book was published in 1919 promoting white supremacy. This was to be achieved by the "Nordic race" being purified through a programme of eugenics. It lambasted those in Europe who had permitted black men to serve in any capacity during the war. The author suggested that 'white' solidarity' had been blown away. Moreover, the book continued that the use of black soldiers during the war had undermined the security of the white race, and it suggested that after the war black and other non-white people needed to be put in subservient positions. This provided more momentum to spread the virus of both direct and institutional racism.

Olusoga and Visram related that after the end of WWI there was much competition for employment. There were calls from the wider public and unions to dismiss Africans, African-Caribbeans, Arabs, Chinese, Filipinos, Greeks, and Somalian people from their employment and replace them by demobilised white men. Similarly, women who worked in factories were also told to return to their domestic roles. Furthermore, white sailors who worked alongside black and other minority seamen during the war told their employers that they were not willing to work alongside their non-European counterparts. This led to many employers dismissing black and other men who were not white. It became clear to this group of soldiers and seamen that these non-white people were not British citizens. They were seen as aliens and viewed with suspicion. Over and above being made unemployed many Black, Chinese, Arabs, Filipinos, Greeks, Somalis and Indians were frequently attacked by white sailors, soldiers, and the locals. These scenes were repeated in Glasgow, South Shields, and London's docklands. Disorders were assisted by fascists in Newport, Tiger Bay in Cardiff, Hull, and Liverpool. Hostels and homes where black and other minorities lived were ransacked and looted. Most of these perpetrators were white people from other parts of Europe. They joined in the attacks even though they were not British and had no connection to the Empire. The police, according to Olusoga, were either unable or unwilling to intervene, but when they did, they raided some of the hostels where black soldiers and other minority seamen stayed. All these actions culminated to the 1919 race riots. Black, Chinese, Arabs, Filipinos, Greeks, Somalis and Indians were accused of lowering standards, undercutting wages, taking white peoples' jobs, had poor morals, and were seen as a threat. Efforts were made to provide financial inducement for these men to go back to their countries. However, this failed.

The contributions of Indians in WWI (1914-1918)

According to Visram, India being part of the British Empire was automatically involved in the war and Tharoor, (2017) (8) stated Mahatma Gandhi supported the war. Indians had contributed significantly to Britain's imperial past before WWI. They were battle hardened by regular wars against among others the Mughal Empire. These soldiers were mainly from Punjab, the Northwest Frontier, Rajasthan, the hills of Garhwal and Nepal and were known as so-called 'martial races'. Visram added that various Indian troops loaded ammunition, chopped trees, built airports and roads, and provided medical staff and hospital ships. Help was also provided in monetary form. India gave Britain £100 million and between £20 to £30 million in the following war years. Both Tharoor and Visram agreed that when the war started Britain had no mass army or conscription, so the well-trained Indian soldiers were available to cover the shortfall. Morton-Jack (2023) (9) instanced that more than 1.5 million Indians enlisted for the British in 1914. Visram posited that this was the first time Indian soldiers were fighting on the European soil. They fought in all major theatres of war on land, air, and sea along British troops. In 1914 the British Expeditionary Force had been wiped out so the Indian soldiers filled the void. This is supported by Tharoor, who estimated the number of Indian soldiers to be around 1.2 million sent abroad and the casualty number of around 101,439 soldiers. In Europe, Indian soldiers were among the first victims who suffered the horrors of the trenches. Many were killed in droves before the war reached its second year and others in ill-judged military manoeuvres. This raised the likelihood that Indians were used as cannon fodder. Many soldiers were thrust into unfamiliar lands, harsh conditions, cold climates, and against unknown enemies. The Indian soldiers were provided with rifles which were no match against the Germans with superior weapons, which explained the high number of Indian casualties. However, they stopped the German's advance on a number of fronts, and their contribution cannot be dismissed.

Finnigan, (2018) (10) stated the Indian soldiers were treated very well regarding maintaining cultural traditions and meeting dietary needs. By contrast, Visram related Indian soldiers were exposed to the inhumanity of Christianity and shocked that many dead bodies were left on the battlefield after they were killed by enemy forces. Most Indian soldiers were very badly treated, lost hope of getting off the battlefield alive, and morale was very low. They were segregated and paid less than their white counterparts and had different terms of service. Some Indian soldiers rebelled, and in some cases committed self-harm. Visram continued that Indian soldiers were sent into the combat zone first, with the white British soldiers following later. Although Indian soldiers developed a glowing reputation in the war, there was a view they were very good but had to be led by white officers. Indians were not allowed to be officers or train with white British soldiers. Visram posited that the reason for not being promoted to officers was that the Indians were "not of pure European stock" and that British soldiers would not take orders from Indian officers. Indians also faced discrimination in their hour of need as English nurses could not treat Indian soldiers. The nurses' role was supervisory. The Indian soldiers questioned why they were able to fight for the country but not to be cared for by white nurses. Consequently, many were left with various forms of injuries and were not able to reach India for treatment. Barracks were like prisons, with security guards and surrounded by fences. One of the rational for the segregated barracks was to keep white women away from Indian soldiers. Tharoor cited a series of occasions when Indian troops were dispatched overseas to protect British interests and paid by Indian funds. There were deployments of the Indian army to China, Ethiopia, Malaya, Malta, Egypt, Somaliland, Sudan, South Africa, and Tibet. Furthermore, every British soldier posted in India was paid, equipped, and fed, and eventually pensioned by the Indian government. Even then there were significant disparities in the rank, pay, promotion, pensions, amenities, and rations between the European and Indian soldiers. In addition to soldiers, Tharoor posited India's labour and commercial skills helped cement imperial rule abroad. All these were never acknowledged or even compensated for the families they left behind. This form of discrimination continued. For example, in the Indian Civil service, most applicants were turned down with only a handful appointed to lower grades. They had positions but no real authority. It only changed when WWI drove thousands of young British men to officer duty in the trenches rather than in the service that the British grudgingly realised the need to recruit more Indian officers but still with no real authority.

The contribution of black African, African-Caribbean, and Indian soldiers was and remain largely ignored. Once the war was over, they were neglected by the British with and for whom they had fought. Many Indians were also ignored by their own country and it was argued they were fighting for the very same empire that was oppressing them. In return for India's extraordinary support, the British had promised to deliver a progressive self-rule at the end of the war. This promise was not fulfilled. India was failed at an economic and political level.

Back in Britain, Sherwood, (2018) (11) expanded, more Indians fought with the British from 1914 to 1918 than the combined total of Australian, New Zealand, Canadian, and South African troops. Some 34,000 Indian soldiers were killed on battlefields in Europe, Africa, and the Middle East; but the part they played in the war has been whitewashed from history. The colonial masters repaid their bravery and sacrifices with brutality and prejudice, or more poignantly with racism. 1000 veteran interview testimonies from the British Empire's First World War Indian servicemen have been offered to the British Library. These first-hand accounts paint a picture of racial segregation and discrimination alongside extraordinary bravery and an awakening hunger for civil rights and independence. One interviewed said: "We were slaves." He spoke of a "curtain of fear" separating the Indian and white soldiers. The Indian soldiers were subject to floggings and other inhumane physical punishment, paid less than their white counterparts, segregated in camps and on trains and ships, denied home leave, and barred from positions of command. Finnigan, asserted Indian hospitals, burial grounds and memorials were hastily built in Brighton England for the wounded, but many felt that their movement was curtailed, and they were treated like prisoners. Visram related that after the 1919 uprising, there were determined efforts by the Home Office to consider repatriate all the unemployed coloured seamen. If this did not take place these soldiers would face destitution, may become desperate, and become a threat to public order. Many long-term residents with British passports or other documentation were still viewed as aliens. Moreover, passports were seized, and the individuals were given inducements to return to their countries of origin.

Contribution of Black Africans and African-Caribbean's during WWII (1939-1945)

According to Parsons (2015) (12), approximately one million sub-Saharan Africans served in some capacity during the Second World War. On the civilian front, even more African women and men produced vast quantities of food and strategic materials for the Allied war effort. The impact of the war on the lives of ordinary people throughout the African continent was therefore unquestionably profound and substantial. They fought alongside the British, French, Belgium, and Italian troops and contributed to the war effort. Buchanan (2020) (13) and BBC (14) indicated that from 1939-1945, some 15,000 African soldiers lost their lives fighting for Britain. Much like their European comrades, African servicemen put their lives at risk to fight for the freedom of the West. Those not engaged in active combat greased the war machine by becoming labourers, porters, carriers, cooks, and mechanics. African servicemen received training in mechanical work, carpentry, and joinery. They learned how to use mortars and machine guns, became signalmen, drivers, and medical orderlies. In 2019, Brown reported a document was found in the British archives that revealed African soldiers who served in the British Army during WWII were paid three times less than their white counterparts. Several MPs requested an official enquiry, and Lord Richard Dannatt, former head of the British Army, suggested that the government consider compensation for the veterans impacted by the inequality. No enquiry was held. As regards to West Indians, more than 10,000 crossed the Atlantic Ocean in response to the call of joining the war efforts. Some paid their own fare, worked in Lancashire factories, airfields in Kent, and forests in the Scottish Highlands. African-Caribbeans provided fundamental support to the war effort. Similarly, during the First World War they felt they had a duty to answer the call from the mother country. The push factor was the serious economic situation and a powerful hurricane in the West Indies itself. In a similar vein to World War I, African-Caribbeans were again attacked and chased while walking in Liverpool streets and had their houses damaged and looted. Their contributions to the war, Parsons, Brown, and BBC all concurred that as in WWI, was whitewashed from literature and history. It took individuals and researchers to investigate and bring the African-Caribbeans contribution to the fore. The whitewashing was deliberate, intentional, and implemented with military precision. Fryer posits the active discrimination and racism continued. Direct racism was supported by institutional racism, and it took several forms, demonstrably attacks by white people and communities. Institutional racism was illustrated by support of these attacks from the British authorities who ignored the gross insults meted out to black and other minority military personnel. Other soldiers and seamen were complicit when some firms either flatly refused to take on "coloured" men or put endless obstacles in their way with the expectation they would seek employment elsewhere.

Black Americans in Britain during WWII

Imperial War Museum (IWM) (no date) (15) revealed during the Second World War, American servicemen and women were posted to Britain to support Allied operations in the Northwest Europe. Between January and December 1942, about 1.5 million of American service personnel landed on British shores. They would be stationed all over UK, particularly in rural areas to support the US Army Air Force. About

150,000 were black and were consigned to supply and service roles. These black Americans were warmly received by the British public but faced open hostilities from their own white countrymen and were segregated in role and accommodation. The War Department (of USA) isolated black troops into all black units and provided them with separate training and accommodation. The British government was uneasy about the segregation policy of the USA but felt they needed to keep on good terms with the American government. To this end, the British government advised the local population not to get too friendly with the black Americans. IWM reported that many business owners (shops and pubs) refused to serve the black Americans for fear of reprisals in the form of losing custom from most of the white soldiers. Nonetheless, many white local girls dated the black soldiers, and this caused even more angst among the authorities. This was used as another pretext to attack and alienate black Americans.

WWII and the contribution of Indians

The involvement of Indians was interlinked with the battle of the independence of India. Chandra (1989) (16) posited that when the War started, Indians in Bombay held an anti-war protest and this was followed by strikes in parts of India; much to the disgust of the British government. Initially India was very reluctant to join the Allied forces. They saw it as another way to serve the imperialist Britain and not for peace or democracy. Indians were of the view that they could not support imperialism. India could not fight for freedom of others while they were still enslaved. Some members of the Indian Congress saw the British stand against fascism amounted to hypocrisy as Britain itself was responsible for blatant human rights violations in the colonies. For Indians, many famines and the Jallianwala Bagh massacre in 1919 were in the forefront of their minds. The Indian Congress was debating their stand between non-violence as proposed by Gandhi or other strategies of involvement. Pacific Atrocities Education (2020) (17) suggested that there were discussions for India to form a military alliance with either Germany or Japan to secure independence from Britain. After lengthy discussion with various British representatives, an agreement was reached that India would be given a dominion status if India helped in the war against fascism. The British had other ideas; they took India into the war without any consultation (Fisher, 1997) (18). Within India the mood also changed when fascists were winning in Europe and Japan was making rapid advances and nearing India itself.

Gee (2020) (19) instanced that 2.5 million people from the British Raj fought against the Axis powers. Whilst some Indians were loyal to Britain, those who signed up were encouraged by offerings of payment through food, land, money, and sometimes technical or engineer training. Many were desperate for work. During the First World War, despite the Bengal famine in 1943 which killed at least three million people, Indian hierarchy provided around £100 million to the War fund (Visram). As WWII progressed, the British relaxed the requirements for sign-ups in India, and even underweight or anaemic applicants were granted positions in the forces. This illustrated the British desperation for men. Pacific Atrocities Education pointed out that those Indian soldiers fought throughout the world. This included in the European theatre against Germany, and the South Asian regions defending the territory against the Japanese in Burma (now Myanmar). India provided the largest volunteer force of any nation during WWII; their participation was crucial to the victory of the allied forces and liberated Italy from Nazi control. The Indian divisions led the advance to the Battle of Monte Casino. Pacific Atrocities Education, however, reported despite all their contributions most Indian officers faced discrimination at the hands of their fellow British officers and were often viewed as outcasts. They were also often paid less and had to endure harsher conditions than their British counterparts. Even the famous multi-million-pound film *Dunkirk* failed to depict the contribution of Indian soldiers during the battle. Visram argued that most of the contributions made by Indians in both World Wars (like the African and African-Caribbean contribution) have been written out of history. Very few have any memorial to commemorate their invaluable contribution. It is possible to suggest that these were intentional strategies, as they do not align with the idea that these wars were 'white and European wars'. Churchill boasted that British people "stood alone" against Hitler, but it was all about reinforcing the ideology of white superiority and giving more credence to racism.

The Chinese seamen

Parliament, House of Commons (2021) (20), and a Labour MP from Riverside (Liverpool) made a searing speech in the House of Parliament on 21st July 2021. This date, according to Johnson, is significant as it marked the 75th anniversary of the forced deportation by the Home Office of thousands of Chinese seamen who served in the Allied war effort. They put their lives on the line in enemy waters to support the British war effort in its hour of need by keeping Britain fed, fuelled and safe. They manned ships and brought food and arms from the USA. During the war as many as 20,000 Chinese seamen worked in the shipping industry out of the Liverpool docks. They were very badly treated, only receiving half the basic wages compared to their British crewmates and on worse terms and conditions. These men did the most dangerous jobs in the engine rooms and worked below decks. However, they were not granted the standard £10 a month war risk bonus, and as a reward for their bravery, when they died in battle their families and loved ones received less compensation. Thousands gave their lives during the perilous campaign under heavy bombardment from Nazi U-boats. Grimsditch (2022) (21) provided graphic pictures of the squalid condition in Liverpool hotels where they lived. The images showed the intolerable conditions as these men washed in sinks and buckets, and cooked food in stoves in their dingy rooms, and slept on bunk beds. By the end of the Second World War, the Home Office estimated there were around 2,000 decommissioned Chinese seamen. The war survivors returned to Liverpool, where many had formed relationships with local women. They set up homes and started families, but from late 1945, unbeknown to the Chinese seamen, moves were afoot to forcibly deport them.

In October 1945, Johnson stated the Home Office without consulting the House of Parliament or the House of Lords, and with no information to the press, made a decision. The decision was 'Compulsory repatriation of *undesirable* Chinese seamen'. Allegations were made that they had married prostitutes and had trouble with the police. This was a plan to support the case that these men were *"undesirables"*. Johnson pointed out that there was no evidence to substantiate any of these allegations. Nonetheless, Chinese men were subsequently rounded up by police and immigration officers prowling the streets. A number were snatched from their homes and dumped unceremoniously in countries they left decades ago. Families themselves believed that their husbands or fathers simply deserted them, and some died never knowing the truth. It is estimated that two thousand men were forcibly deported by the Home Office, which only became apparent after official records Home Office 213/926 became known. As a result, children began to gain an insight into what went on. Details were sketchy and incomplete leaving some still searching for answers. These details were captured by many of the families of the men who were subject to this appalling crime. There were calls for an enquiry and apology but to date it is unclear if any of these were offered.

The Polish Resettlement Act 1947

While black African, African-Caribbean, Asian, Arab, Filipino, Somali, Greek and Chinese people were being actively and systematically discriminated against while in and out of the armed forces, the government was involved in another activity. The activity involved not only the Polish but other eastern European army personnel from Ukraine and Latvia. According to Blaszczyk (no date) (22), after the end of WWII, it became clear that Polish forces and refugees abroad would not be able to return to their homeland. This was due to the Nazi-Soviet pact. Germany claimed Western Poland and part of Lithuania; the Soviet Union was to occupy Eastern Poland, the Baltic States and part of Finland. The pact did not last long. Over one million Poles were displaced, including armed forces, prisoners of war, refugees, and survivors of forced labour and concentration camps. They were afraid that if they returned to Poland they would be seen as enemies of the new Communist regime and imprisoned or even shot (My Learning) (23). The Polish had fought alongside the British forces in the same way that the Africans, African-Caribbeans, Indians, and Chinese serviced the war ships. Blaszczyk indicated the British government took responsibility for some Polish people. Soldiers and airmen serving overseas were to be helped through the Corps to stay in the United Kingdom and settle into civilian life. Service in the Corps was intended to be an opportunity for retraining and education; it was agreed with the British trade unions that prospective Polish employees could only be recruited from the Polish Resettlement Corps (PRC) and would be placed in 'approved' Ministry of Labour jobs. They received help in education to aid them settle and merge the Polish and British cultures. Olusoga elaborated that the Polish and their families who previously lived in Britain and served in the war were given the right to settle permanently. It is estimated that between 150,000-220,000 members of the Polish forces and their families were the beneficiaries. Parliament, House of Parliament (1947) (24) indicated other forms of assistance were offered via pensions and allowance for widows. A further 80,000 Ukrainians, and Latvians were also recruited under the European workers Scheme. The end of the war and the reluctance to return to their home countries functioned as push factors, while the need for expansion of the British labour force served as a pull factor. It is acknowledged by the authors above that they all made significant contribution to the war and the subsequent rebuilding of Britain. The treatment and reception of the Polish, Ukrainians and Latvians differed markedly with the way Black Africans, African-Caribbeans, Chinese, Arabs and other non-white people was plain to see. Nonetheless, there was still resentment to the presence of Polish and other European people, and many were directed towards jobs the local people would not do.

Conclusion

There are recurring themes in the way Black Africans, African-Caribbeans, Indians, Chinese and other servicemen were treated before, during, and after both World Wars. They were segregated, discriminated against, paid less than their white counterparts, harassed and attacked by their fellow 'colleagues', the police, and members of the public. Many were chased by members of the local community for simply walking along the streets. They had their houses and hostels attacked resulting in considerable damage. Others were killed or executed. No one came to their rescue. They were refused service in pubs and clubs as owners were left in no doubt by the white soldiers that they would withdraw their custom if these venues accommodated black service men. After the end of the Second World War the government was determined to employ white foreign workers to fill the ever-growing demand for workers. Employers and white workers were determined not to employ or work alongside Black Africans, West Indians, and Indians, and attacked them when they challenged the colour bar. This was in stark contrast to the way Polish soldiers and their families were treated. In keeping with the government plan to employ white foreigners instead of black British citizens, Polish soldiers were offered employment, education, and a pension. The government, Olusoga stated, actively discouraged the employment of Black Africans and African-Caribbeans. They went as far as informing the African and Caribbean governments (in their respective countries) that there were no employment opportunities in Britain. This, given the fact that many Africans, Indians, and African-Caribbeans, were British as they were all from British colonies. This was of no significance to the British authorities. Black African, African-Caribbean, Indian, and Chinese people were of less value compared to their Polish and other Eastern European counterparts. The colour of their skin took precedence over their citizenship. All these were rooted in the belief that white people were superior, and the government not only reflected but reinforced this ideology. It could be argued that the Poles and other Eastern Europeans had their countries devastated after the WWII and this was the antecedent for the government to act. However, the British inflicted much poverty in Africa, African-Caribbean countries and India during the days when colonialism was at its height. This caused another slow war. As Gandhi said, "poverty is the worst form of violence." Furthermore, most of the contributions from African, African-Caribbean, Indian and Chinese soldiers and seamen during the war were whitewashed from British history. In the final analysis they fought for the freedom for white Europeans not theirs. Europeans were free to continue to oppress their Black, Asian, and Chinese counterparts with help from the governments of any political persuasion. These are illustrations that direct and institutional racism were well-established. The above discussion highlighted the aftermath of WWI and WWII, The next chapter discusses the long presence of Black and Asian people in Britain since 1555.

CHAPTER 6
AN OVERVIEW OF THE PRESENCE OF BLACK AFRICAN, AFRICAN-CARIBBEAN, AND ASIAN PEOPLE IN BRITAIN

This chapter provides a snapshot of the presence of Black and Asian people in Britain. It discusses how they arrived, their experiences and contribution to the economic, social and cultural life in Britain. This provides an insight into a part of British history and places contemporary events in a wider context. Much of the inequalities and racism discussed are rooted in British history and have implications for all its institutions. This includes the NHS. The discussion is presented in two main sections. The experiences of Africans and African-Caribbeans are outlined, followed by the experiences of Asian peoples.

Black African and African-Caribbean people

A recent facial reconstruction of a 10,000-year-old skeleton called the "Cheddar Man" was found in Gough's Cave in Cheddar Gorge, Somerset, England. It revealed a man with bright blue eyes, slightly curly hair, and dark skin. Technological advances led scientists to identify that the ancient DNA proved he is genetically like other dark-skinned individuals from the Mesolithic era[9]. The DNA was found in people from Spain, Hungary, and Luxemburg. Their DNA has already

---

[9] An approximate period of between 10,000-7,000 BC when man invented tools for hunting and collection of food.

been sequenced. The new revelation placed the Cheddar Man among a group of hunter-gatherers that are thought to have migrated to Europe at the end of the last Ice Age some 11,000 years ago. The name was given as he was found in Cheddar Gorge in Somerset (Gibbens 2018) (1). It is estimated that around 10 per cent of indigenous British ancestry can be linked to that population and that the British population was completely replaced by incoming farmers around 6,000 years ago (University College London) (UCL 2018) (2). This view chimes with Rutherford (2020) (3) who opined that the earliest members of our species can be traced in what is now Morocco around 300,000 years ago. Rutherford suggested humans are starting to think that in the beginning we came from a pan-African species, a mixture of diverse populations from around that mighty continent. Early humans, he continued, migrated into Asia and Europe within the last quarter of a million years. Fryer (1991) (4) indicated there were African people in Britain before the English came. The former were soldiers in the Roman Imperial Army that occupied the southern part of the island for three and a half centuries. They were among the troops defending Hadrian's Wall in third century AD and was a division of the Moors named after Marcus Aurelius. The latter was originally raised in North Africa and his unit was based near Carlisle. An African soldier is reputed to have reached Britain about the year 210. There were traces of an African presence in the British Isle about 400-500 years after the Romans left (Fryer). Furthermore, about four hundred Black Tudors were present during 1500 to 1640.

In the seventeenth and eighteenth centuries thousands of black youngsters were brought to Britain against their will as domestic slaves. Others came of their own accord and stayed for a while or settled here. Fryer noted that between 1562-1563, John Hawkins was the first English man to line his pockets by trafficking in black slaves on the first English triangular journey. He acquired at least three hundred inhabitants of the Guinea coast. By 1570 English merchants were trafficking slaves in a really organised way. African slaves were brought by these merchants and were sent to North America and the West Indies. Towards the end of the sixteenth century, it was beginning to be a smart thing for titled and propertied families in England to have a black slave or two among the household servants. Many of the slaves were gifted musicians and entertainers. No matter how entertaining they were for the owners and the Royal family, it did not cut any ice with Queen Elizabeth I. In 1596 she sent letters to mayors of London and other towns asking them to expel these blackamoores; as there were already "too many of them" and they were "taking food out of *her* subjects' mouths". This coincided with a bad harvest. Furthermore, these blackamoores were to be avoided as they were infidels and had no understanding of Christ or his gospel. Fryer argued, several attempts were made to deport them but they failed. Therein lays the challenge of the frequently held maxim that hostility was or is due to the size of the Black or Asian population. Firstly, there were Black people in Britain before the English came, and Africans and Asians and their descendants have been living in Britain for close on to five hundred years. Secondly there were very few Black or Asian people in Britain at that time. The population at that time was around three million and the Black and Asian population around 10,000. Whether the deportation took place or not is immaterial, it was the ideology which underpinned her actions and the blame attached to the blackamoores. They were allegedly "taking food out of *her* subjects' mouths".

The slave trade continued and by 1660-1689 fifteen of London's mayors and twenty-five of the sheriffs were shareholders in the Royal African Company, as were 38 of the City's Aldermen between 1672 and 1690. London, and Liverpool were deeply immersed in the slave trade. Olusoga (2016) (5) pointed out that Bristol, Cardiff, Manchester,

Glasgow, London and other minor ports grew very rich on the back of the slave trade. In 1729 a merchant summarised the contemporary view:

"our trade with Africa is very profitable to the Nation in general; it has this Advantage, that it carries no Money out, and not only supplies our Plantation with Servants, but brings in a great Deal of Bullion for those who are sold to the Spanish West-Indies. The supplying our Plantations with Negros is of that extraordinary Advantage to us, that the Planting, Sugar and Tobacco, and carrying on Trade there could not be supported without [t]hem; which Plantations... are the great Cause of the Increase of the Riches of the Kingdom...All this increase of our Treasure proceeds chiefly from the Labour of Negros in the Plantation".

Fryer continued, gradually the English were "becoming habituated" to slavery and "caused liberty-loving Englishmen no serious searching of conscience". By 1780, no black slaves meant no sugar and rum punch. Increase for these products had risen exponentially and slave owners were making 'bricks of gold'. During the same time in London, Bristol, and Liverpool ships were loaded with muskets, brass, rods, cutlery and other materials from various parts of England. They were used to barter for slaves on the African coasts. The slaves were shipped across the Atlantic and the notorious middle passage. There is general agreement that the profits for the evil trade in slavery led to the industrial revolution in Britain. (Fryer, Olusoga, Williams (1944) (6) and Doyal and Pennell (1979) (7).

Many slaves did not tolerate the savage and gratuitous maltreatment, many uprisings occurred, and most were brutally put down by the power and the armoury of slave owners. Two examples are summarised: Rallying calls for freedom, equality and brotherhood was active in Paris and this idea found its way to the island of St Domingue (now Haiti) which was under French control. In 1791, half a million people of African descent who toiled in chains rose to seize their freedom. It was the largest rebellion in history and was the only one that was successful during that period. The 'victory' had two consequences. First, it confirmed in the minds of slave owners that slaves were able to restrain their supposedly innate violence, and second it consolidated resistance of any talk of abolition. The other uprising was in Morant Bay in Jamaica. Olusoga argued that the Morant Bay war remains an open wound and a burning grievance to this day. It was a brutal retaliation to skirmishes which led to disproportionately severe repression, summary executions, and punishment for transgressors. The American Civil war provided some impetus, and a crowd of local black people marched the streets of Morant Bay. They attacked the police station, took possession of some arms, and confronted the local militia. The uprising did not spread any further. Blood had been spilt, including that of white people, government property was destroyed, and the law had been contravened. The reaction was swift and uncompromising. Olusoga related how for six weeks the West India Regiment accompanied by the local militia was let loose upon the parish of St Thomas with its capital being Morant Bay. They were assisted by additional troops and martial law was imposed. The operation ended up with 439 black Jamaicans killed, six were dragged from their homes, six hundred men and women caught by the troops were flogged and some men were lashed with wire whips. Over a thousand homes were burnt and people who had worked themselves out of absolute poverty were made destitute and penniless.

Asians in Britain
Fryer posited that some black servants and entertainers in Britain during the eighteenth century were Mohammedans and Hindus. Most

came from Bengal, Madras, and elsewhere in India. It is also well-known that the English and French in their wars in India used Africans as cannon fodder and engaged in slavery in other parts of Africa. Having Black and/or Asian servants was seen as a status symbol and many Englishwomen who travelled to India brought Asian servants with them. Like most African slaves in Britain, Asians were sometimes ill-treated, and some ran away and were the subject of advertising as a method of notifying the escape and ensuring their return. Furthermore, Asian slaves were sometimes advertised for sale, while free Asians occasionally advertised their availability for work. Tharoor (2016) (8) cited work by Durant who referred to India as

"The British conquest of India was the invasion and destruction of a high civilisation by a trading company (the British East India Company) utterly without scruple or principle, careless of art and greedy of grain, over-running with fire and sword a country temporarily disordered and helpless, bribing and murdering, annexing and stealing, and beginning that career of illegal and "legal" plunder which has now gone on ruthlessly for one hundred and seventy years".

Tharoor expanded by noting that the British took advantage of the collapse of the Mughal Empire and the rise of several warring groups contending for authority across eighteenth-century India. The British had subjugated vast lands through the power of their artillery and the cynicism of their amorality. He maintained the British displaced the Nawabs (aristocrats) and Maharajas (Kings) and emptied their treasuries, and stripped farmers of their own lands they had tilled for generations. Tharoor referred to Madison's work who revealed that at the beginning of the eighteenth-century India's share of the world economy was 23 per cent as large as all of Europe put together. By the time the British departed India, it had dropped to just 3 per cent. The reason Tharoor stated, was because India was governed for the benefit of Britain. Its rise for two hundred years was financed by its depredations in India. All was made possible through the East India Company founded in London in 1599. In India, the company built new trading bases in Calcutta, Madras, and Bombay and by the mid-eighteenth century it generated at least an eighth of Britain's import trade (Tharoor). While Britain was getting rich, India and Indians were not only suffering but dying from a series of famines during British rule. These were the Great Bengal Famine in 1770, Madras in 1782-83, and Chalisa Famine in Delhi and the surrounding areas. The fatality figures are horrifying. From 1700 to 1900, Tharoor estimated that twenty-five million Indians died in famines including 15 million in the five famines in the second half of the nineteenth century.

There were other atrocities committed by the British. One was the Jallianwala Bagh massacre in 1919. Tharoor detailed the events before, during, and after the massacre. A few days prior to the massacre the British government arrested two nationalist leaders in the Punjab. Some minor disturbances followed. The police retaliated and killed ten demonstrators. This resulted in troops being sent to Amritsar. General Reginald Dyer was in charge of these troops and on that day he became aware that a crowd of some 10,000-15,000 Indians gathered in the park. A notice of meeting prohibition was declared but it was not clear if those who gathered were aware of it. As far as they were concerned they were there peacefully celebrating the Sikh festival of Baisakhi. The General arrived at the park via the one and only narrow entrance, and without ordering for the crowd to disperse and without firing a warning shot; he ordered his troops to fire at the crowd with specific instructions to aim at the "thickest" part. The crowd started to scream and tried to escape, but Dyer ordered his men to keep firing until all the ammunition was exhausted. When they had finished, the troops had used 1,650 rounds and killed 379 people (according to the British).

The unofficial number was 1499 people. There are also reports that after the shooting the only gate to the park was locked. This prevented families and other people to help the wounded or remove the deceased. Furthermore, an investigation conducted by the Indian Congress suggested that many Indians who were outside the park had been ordered by the British to crawl on their bellies. The official commission on inquiry whitewashed Dyer's conduct and was regarded by British imperialists as 'The Man Who Saved India'. Although he was subsequently removed from his duties, Dyer retired on a handsome pension. Sandbrook (2019) (9) reported that one Sikh man was determined to avenge this massacre. He located and shot the elderly Dyer on 13th March 1940 in London two decades later. This has been well reported in India but less so in Britain. The Jallianwala Bagh massacre provided more ammunition and helped galvanise India's cause for independence. This was achieved in 1947 but with the British inspired partition of India. Unfortunately, there were very serious ideological differences between Mahatma Gandhi and his counterpart Mohamed Ali Jinnah and this was exploited to the full by the British authorities. Muslims who were a substantial part of India's population after collaboration between Muslim leaders and the British they decided to have their states. Much blood was shed between the Indians and Muslims. Two nations were born because of the partition. They are Pakistan and East Pakistan, now Bangladesh.

The abolition of slavery

The abolition of slavery in 1833 did not begin by a sudden attack of humanity from the stratosphere. There were regular uprisings and the anti-slavery movement began to get more active during the 1769s. According to Fryer, this was led initially by Quaker Anthony Benezet and his writings influenced Thomas Clarkson and Granville Sharp. Other central figures who were instrumental in the abolition movement were the Africans; Otobah Cugoano, Olaudah Equiano, Mary Prince, Elizabeth Heyrick, Hannah More and Sons of Africa. Much support came from all over Britain which culminated in 100 petitions being sent to the House of Parliament in 1788. Thomas (2020) (10) listed seven reasons as to why slavery was finally abolished in Britain: (1) A series of resolutions that called for the improvement of conditions for slaves in His Majesty's colonies were not implemented by planters. (2) Between 1807 and 1833, three of Britain's most valuable Caribbean colonies all experienced violent slave uprisings. The rebellions in the West Indies, accompanied by the brutal suppressions, strengthened abolitionist arguments regarding the instability of the Caribbean dominions. (3) White colonists in the West Indies were always viewed with suspicion from those in the metropolis. They were often disdained for their excessively ostentatious displays of wealth and their gluttonous habits. (4) The economic deterioration of the West Indian colonies led to an over production of sugar and significant reduction in profit. (5) Free labour was a far superior model as it was cheaper, more productive, and efficient. This was proven by the success of the free labour system employed in the East Indies. (6) There was a change in the political environment when it comes to understanding why emancipation occurred. It is no coincidence that slavery was abolished a year after the Great Reform Act of 1832 and there was a subsequent election of a Whig government with liberal ideologies under the leadership of Lord Grey. (7) The abolition of slavery faced several rejections in both Houses of Parliament and was finally abolished in 1833. It did not result in the immediate abolition. Olusoga pointed out that all those who worked in the fields were to continue their labour for an additional six years. The system was euphemistically called "apprenticeship" and it excluded Indian slaves. Its successor was a system of indentured labour. History Hit (no date) (11) defined indentured labour as a system of bonded labour that was instituted following the abolition of slavery. Indentured labourers were recruited to work on sugar, cotton, and tea plantations, and rail construction projects in British colonies in the West Indies, Africa and South East Asia. BBC Culture (2020) (12) elaborated that the slave owners were compensated as a direct result of the abolition of slavery. The slaves were not. The compensation was fully paid in 2015. This meant that British citizens contributed to this settlement. It cannot be ruled out that many BAME people who currently live in and those who left Britain contributed via taxation to settle the compensation claim. In effect BAME people who live or have lived in Britain have contributed to compensating the very people who enslaved their forebears. I witnessed the tail end of indentured labouring in my young days. In the late 1960s, my father occasionally took me to work with him. As a labourer he grew, cut, and harvested sugar cane for the use of Britain and Europe. He worked six days a week in the hot sun, rain, and other weather conditions to cut and load sugar canes trucks. He never had any paid holiday or sick pay. His measly wages were not adequate and had to be supplemented by working our land to keep us fed and watered. I am supposed to be "pleased" that the evil trade has been abolished by taxpayers, not realising the offence it would cause survivors like me. It is difficult to comprehend why I should compensate slave owners when they killed many of my family members. The slaves themselves got nothing. The counter argument would be that indentured labourers were not slaves per se. For those who were duped with advance pay and ripped from their family and country like my forebears to work for pittance, and being continuously abused, it felt like slavery.

After the abolition of the slavery in the British West Indies and after a period of unpaid apprenticeship many liberated Africans left their former masters. This abolition did not include India. Given that the entire slave trade was so well organised it was incredulous that the inclusion of Indians in the abolition movement was overlooked. The abolition of slavery led to a significant drop in manpower. They had a reserve army at their disposal. The sugar planters looked to India. The solution was the hiring of Indians as indentured or contract labourers which in many ways resembled enslavement. Williams asserted that slave trading in the early stages in the New World involved the Indians and not black Africans. Indians rapidly succumbed to the excessive labour demanded of them, the insufficient diet and the white man's disease, and their inability to 'adjust' to a new way of life. The successor of the Indian was in fact the poor whites and with the intention of putting them to industrious work and favoured emigration. These were indentured servants and tenants fleeing the restriction of feudalism. Irish men were seeking freedom from landlords, bishops and Germans were running away from war. Other white people were petty criminals; some were even plied with liquor whilst children were given sweets and told they were off to a new adventure beyond the sea. In the final analysis they did not provide adequate labour, and the planters turned to black Africans again. They were cheaper, plentiful and as quoted "three blacks work better and cheaper than one white man" was a popular view. After the abolition of slavery in the British West Indies, many were unemployed, illiterate and poor.

Indians were duped and transported to various British colonies for an initial five-year period, but very few, if any at all, made it back (Hiro 1991) (13). Most were mistreated just like the black Africans and Indians were treated as inhumanely as the enslaved Africans. They were confined to their states and paid pitiful sums. Any breach of contract was heavily fined. If they did not work they were not paid or fed, they simply starved. Importing contract labour from India was suspended in 1840. The Indian labour market was cut off and some Europeans were recruited thereafter. This failed miserably and the British went back to contracting Indians. This time legislation was passed to protect the well-being of the Indian immigrants. Provisions were made for basic supply provision in housing, food rations, clothing, and wages. All depended on a task completion basis. Indians were held in depots. Many were deceived about work on offer and were hustled into waiting ships, unprepared for long journeys (Mahoney, 2020) (14). Recruitment continued apace and East Indian workers came from all walks of life and with varied skills. Some Indian landowners were forced off their lands when wealthy Britons began to buy smallholdings. Despite the safeguards put in place by Parliament to prevent indentured workers suffering a new form of enslavement, plantation owners continued to abuse these workers. This I witnessed in the 1960s. I have no doubt that my forebears were some of these people who were duped and transported to Mauritius. This part of my father's history is limited. My father never talked about his parents; maybe it was a coping strategy and/or far too painful to bring to the fore. My father toiled all day, in all weathers for measly wages. If he did not go to work due to illness, he would not get paid. Taking a holiday was an alien concept to him. These were replicated to many of my extended family and neighbours. The exhaustion and despair was not only visible but palpable. They were trapped with nowhere to go or turn to. They fought the only way they could and never gave up. Indian slavery in India was formally abolished in 1843 but this contrasts with Akbar's view. At the end of nineteenth century, Mahatma Gandhi argued with the colonial government, and it was through his efforts, and intervention by the Indian government, that the indentured scheme finally came to an end in 1917 (Akbar 2006) (15).

The discussion so far has zoomed in on Black Africans and Indians and it would be reasonable to add the British colonial exploitations in Canada, North America, Australia, and New Zealand. One theme runs through these countries and that is without exception during every colonisation process, the original inhabitants of every single one of these countries were displaced, their land seized, and many were killed or maimed. Women were raped, artefacts and culture destroyed and people were degraded and dehumanised. Without exception they were made to feel like strangers in their homes and country. After trafficking in African slavery for around three hundred years and looting India for around two hundred years Britain became extraordinarily rich (Williams). This is how Britain developed wealth off the back of the transatlantic slave trade. This financed the industrial revolution in Britain and here Williams made a direct link between slavery, capitalism and racism.

Conclusion

This chapter has illustrated that Black Africans and Asians have lived in Britain for five hundred years. The evil trade in slavery and systematic exploitation of the above groups of people lasted for centuries. These were conducted with no regrets, remorse, and no regards to humanity. It was an absolute demonstration of the 'superiority' of the white race upon others. Britain got extremely rich and left those exploited people and countries in abject poverty. British rule not only resulted in poverty but was an extreme example of systematic exploitation and dehumanisation of millions of Africans, African-Caribbeans, Indians, and others in the British colonies. Numerous historians and politicians have overlooked this historical account. After the abolition of slavery in 1833, the slave owners were granted compensation. This payment was completed in 2015, and it transpired that BAME citizens have paid taxes and some of which have been used to compensate the very people who killed many members of their family. The suffering, personal distress and trauma continued. The abolition of slavery led the British authorities to turn to India for cheap labour in the shape of another form of bonded labourers. This was abolished in 1843. After providing an overview of the presence of BAME people and their treatment in Britain, the context within which BAME people and 'race' has been placed. The next chapter discusses recent events that continue to adversely impact on BAME people. These are the austerity measures, its impact on inequalities, determinants of health, the NHS, and the life chances of BAME people.

CHAPTER 7
AUSTERITY, ITS IMPACT ON INSTITUTIONS AND BAME PEOPLE

Wilkinson and Picket (2010) (1) provided a broad perspective on how to improve our quality of life. They support the view that for thousands of years the best way to improve our quality of life is to raise material living standards. However, Britain in 2010 was (among mostly European) the fourth largest country with the widest income gap between the rich and the poor. Singapore, the USA, and Portugal were the leading countries. An undated statement by Equality Trust (2) suggested that UK's five richest families now own more wealth than the bottom thirteen million people, and the richest 1 per cent of people in the UK owns the same wealth as 80 per cent of the population. These are reflective of a society that is very hierarchical as the rich and powerful are at the very top and can get the best houses in very pristine locations, best facilities, disposable income, and consequently the best life chances. Another form of inequality has always been the North South divide. The life chances of those living in the North of Britain are and have been markedly much less than those in the South. The gap is also reflected within countries, especially in regional inequalities that resulted in significant health and social problems. Politicians have been very keen to tell us that millions of pounds have been allocated to the NHS, but Wilkinson and Pickett argued that there is no relationship between the amount of health spending per person and life expectancy. They suggested an even distribution of wealth improves the nation's health. In Britain, these have been getting progressively worse. The main reason was the introduction of the austerity measures. This chapter provides an overview of how austerity is having an adverse effect on regional inequalities, determinants of health, and disproportionately impact on the health of BAME people.

In 2008 the global financial system experienced its biggest shock in a century. According to Singh (2024) (3) this was not entirely unexpected. He noted this was years in the making as the financial markets ignored that the days of cheap lending was over and continued to provide loans with little due process. The crash pushed the world's banking system to the brink of collapse. Others argued that this was caused by the lack of regulation in the financial sector. It caused one of the world's biggest financial institutions to be bankrupt and an estimated £90 billion was wiped off the value of Britain's biggest companies in a single day. The Labour government bailed out the banks with an estimated £500 billon (White, 2015) (4). This was supplemented by quantitative easing which effectively meant printing money. BBC 2, (2022) (5) claimed in May 2009 £125 billion were printed and it reached £200 billion by November 2009. This was an attempt to pump money into the economy and to promote recovery. However, the money went to banks, property markets, and private equity firms. Funds went in the pockets of the super-rich. This resulted in the rich getting richer and little if any money trickled down to the lowest earners. Furthermore, huge multinational companies got away with paying little or no tax. BBC 2 stated the top 1 per cent of the population got richer and 99 percent got almost nothing. This was the precursor to the austerity measures which was implemented in 2010 by the incoming coalition government of the Conservatives and the Liberal Democrats.

Definition of Austerity

Austerity is a campaign of budget cuts that the coalition government began in 2010 in the aftermath of the global financial crisis of 2008 (Mueller, 2019) (6). This was the most crippling economic downturn since the Great Depression. Pettinger (2018) (7) agreed and suggested austerity involved policies to reduce government spending (or higher taxes) to try and reduce government budget deficits, during a period of weak economic growth. This is often associated with higher unemployment and lower economic growth. Corporate Finance Institute, (CFI) (2015) (8) concurred and added austerity measures refer to government policies that aimed to reduce public sector debt. Uncontrolled increases in a country's public debt tend to increase financial instability, and if unchecked can cause recession. Undoubtedly, the working classes would be disproportionately impacted as opposed to the well off. Austerity has also been called as "class war". It referred to individuals from lower social classes who are disproportionately affected by reductions in services, while those who are affluent can insulate themselves from such service cuts.

Elliott and Wintour, (2010) (9) stated the government set out to reduce the economic deficit as quickly as possible by reducing welfare costs and 'wasteful' spending. There was a preference for cuts over wealth accumulation via taxation. The then Chancellor announced a £40 billion tax rise, welfare cuts and in Whitehall spending. There is no doubting that this was purely a political decision. CFI indicated that many economists believe austerity as a policy is ineffective as a reduction in government expenditure including cuts in welfare services, health care programmes, and other essential government provided services. Austerity measures tend to affect low wage earners. Thus, the section of society that needs the most assistance during a period of economic instability is harmed the most by austerity-based policies. The British Association of Social Workers (BASW) (2017) (10), whose members deal with the implications of austerity first-hand, agreed. It argued debt reduction is a flawed concept as it creates unemployment, homelessness, inequality, and misery upon the lives of citizens. Reducing expenditure combined with tax reduction for the wealthy reduces state income and fails to achieve balanced economies. It could also be argued that much of the adverse impact of the coalition government came years after the implementation of the austerity measures. This, however, could well have been predicted before using the previous examples and the experience of ordinary people in different countries. In fact, McKee, Karanikolos, and Stuckler (2012) (11) noted that by contrast, the USA's response to the severe financial crisis was not austerity but launched a fiscal stimulus. The result was clear. The American economy is growing and those in Europe, including the UK, are stagnating and struggling to repay rising debts.

A United Nations Committee of independent experts recently issued a harshly worded report on the extent to which public authorities have been complying with international law on socio-economic rights. The Committee monitors state compliance with the International Covenant on Economic, Social and Cultural Rights, which the UK has voluntarily ratified along with 163 other countries (Casla, Burton, and Donald) (2016)(12). The Office of the High Commission for Human Rights (OHCHR 2008) (13) clarified what the covenant entails: They relate to the workplace, social security, family life, participation in cultural life and access to housing, food, water, healthcare, and education. Work should be free from forced labour, with fair wages, and equal pay for equal work. There ought to be limited working hours, safe working environments and freedom to join unions. This is supplemented by Social Security provision in the event of unemployment, sickness, inability to work or old age, right to married life, maternity and paternity protection for families and children. Despite all the evidence of the consequences of austerity measures and the legal requirements, the coalition government opted to reduce national spending by a monumental scale.

Austerity measures have exacerbated long-standing and entrenched inequalities. Significant financial cuts have had a detrimental effect on every determinant of health. Indeed, McKee et al pointed out that austerity has not only been an economic failure, but also a health failure with increasing numbers of suicides and, where cuts in health budgets are being imposed, increasing numbers of people unable to access care. In the UK, the health budget was protected but the significant financial cuts in organisations like the Local Authorities inhibited them to address the social determinants of health. Housing and social care provision being just two examples. This resulted in an increased use of the NHS. Drawing on historical and contemporary evidence, specific reference is made to highlighting how austerity has adversely impacted the lives of BAME people. Furthermore, politicians have exploited inequalities created by austerity to promote anti-immigrant ambiance and were very well supported by sections of the media. It all culminated in BAME people being blamed and held responsible for creating these inequalities. These were explicit especially during the European Referendum. The values and attitudes that were displayed during the slavery days and World Wars were always there but now it was very overt.

The impact of austerity in Britain

Given the already existing and entrenched inequalities, Hernandez, (2021) (14) revealed that the austerity programme has eroded social development in the UK. Spending reductions have led to a precarious public sector labour market. The living standards of many public employees deteriorated. This is reflected in changes to household's disposable income, savings, debt, and reliance on food banks. There is robust evidence that different social problems such as homelessness, crime, and child poverty were becoming more severe during austerity years. The Office for National statistics revealed the national debt did not go down during the imposition of austerity. It rose from 2010-2017, declined in 2019, and began to rise again. Gregory, (2021) (15) quoted that austerity in England is linked to more than 50,000 deaths in the period of 2010-2015. Similar finding was made by the British Medical Journal in 2018. House of Lords Library (2023) (16) stated so far by 2020 over 300,000 excess deaths were attributed to austerity. Male life expectancy declined to 79 years while women were down to 82.9 years. There is general agreement that women's mortality has increased and life expectancy improvement was slowing. In relation to Children Services, MacAlister, in GOV.UK (2022) (17), who led the independent review concluded that

"What we have now is a system increasingly skewed to crisis intervention, with outcomes for children that continue to be unacceptably poor and costs continue to rise".

Local Authorities have experienced significant cuts in grants from central government and these have been reflected in reduction of some key services i.e. youth services, community engagement and libraries. They included among others, the police, road maintenance, libraries, courts, prisons and housing assistance for seniors as local governments suffered significant plunge in revenue. Economic and Research Council (2018) (18) argued most agencies also had their budgets significantly cut. Some of the main changes included maximum rents introduced for housing benefits, and child benefit being frozen (rather than rising with inflation). The age limit for people to share a room under the local housing allowance was increased from 25 to 35-years-old. When the Welfare Reform Act 2012 was introduced, and implemented in 2013, it included the Bedroom tax[10]. As a result, social housing tenants lost up to 25 per cent of their benefit if they had a spare room. This was compounded by the acute shortage of smaller properties and resulted in people being 'trapped' in the house allocated to them through no fault of their own. Universal Credit was outlined as a new means-tested benefit that turned benefits for people employed and unemployed into a single package. Further, Personal Independence Payment (PIP) began to replace Disability Living Allowance (DLA) for new claimants. It involved more stringent medical tests and more frequent testing than the DLA, even for life-long conditions. Benefits for households became capped which meant that benefit levels could not be higher than average wages. Tougher penalties were introduced for benefit fraud and limitations in Legal Aid resulted in a fall in the numbers of people getting state-funded help to challenge benefit cases. From April 2014, existing benefit claimants began to be transferred to Universal Credit.

Impact of people

Between 2010 and 2020 Toynbee and Walker (2020) (19) indicated the austerity has destroyed the fabric of society as we know it. Speaking to people on the frontline revealed the ways their lives have changed forever. What occurred in the UK during these times will scar us for the rest of our lives. There are new jobs which are badly paid, and it is not surprising that debt is mountainous and the gap between the rich and poor has widened.

> *"Entrenching high levels of poverty and inflicting unnecessary misery in one of the richest countries in the world".*

---

[10] This meant if there is one spare bedroom and the property is being rented from the council or housing association, then the Housing Benefit or housing costs would be reduced.

They pointed to the worrying fact that the young are now worse off than their parents at their age; home ownership has declined steeply, families are stuck in life-long and at times precarious private renting. Kingsley, (2018) (20) from United Nations stated that efforts by the government to cut state spending were inflicting unnecessary misery. In 2010, the United Nations report highlighted the government has announced more than £30 billion in cuts to welfare payments, housing subsidies and social services, and the British leadership is in 'a state of denial' about the devastation its policies have wrought. The government disputed those findings, but there are signs that social well-being declined under austerity (Oxfam) (2013) (21). The use of food banks almost doubled between 2013 and 2017. In May 2023, it commented that the "explosion in food poverty and its use is a national disgrace". Austerity measures have led to 600,000 children falling into relative poverty. During the same period, the number of children requiring food hand-outs from the Trussell Trust (the country's largest network of food banks) tripled. It is not just the jobless and their families who are suffering. Two-thirds of poor children have at least one parent who works. Murders and robberies have surged to their highest levels in a decade in England and Wales. Some police leaders blamed cutbacks to police forces as staffing across England and Wales has fallen by about 20,000 officers. Others argued that rising crime may be a knock-on effect of austerity cuts to youth and social services, as well as rising social inequality and poverty. Oxfam continued that when all austerity measures are considered, including cuts to public services and changes to tax and welfare, the poorest tenth of the population are by far the hardest hit, seeing a 30 per cent decrease in their net income during the period 2010-2015. By contrast, the richest tenth will have lost the least or experience a 5 per cent fall in their income. Rawlingson (2021) (22) of Joseph Rowntree Foundation agreed and pointed out that low-income families in the UK have experienced several years of particularly weak income at the same level as they were nearly two decades ago. In addition, I in 5 people were living in poverty in 2019-20. It continued, those living in the deepest poverty already face exclusion from the opportunity to live a healthy and fulfilling life. Low-income families have been forced to rely on emergency support and or to cut back on essentials in the face of higher costs arising from having to stay at home during the lockdown. The Institute for Government in October 2022 argued that public services are in a much more fragile position now than in 2010. This is a result of both the first round of austerity and more recently the pandemic. Cuts are therefore likely to be both more damaging and harder to deliver.

In November 2023, the newly appointed Chancellor delivered his Autumn Statement. He increased benefits and housing costs, but according to Trussell Trust even with this boost Universal Credit will not meet the costs of the essentials. People on the lowest incomes are still facing significant challenges, with a rising tide of hunger and debt which has been pushing food banks to breaking point. All these factors would undoubtedly have significant implications for health.

Austerity and BAME people

As discussed in chapter two, three and four, people of BAME ethnicity have been experiencing various form of racism for centuries. These were in the days of colonialism, the two World Wars, and during the 1940's and beyond. In the health field as discussed above, BAME people have been and are still underserved in the health sector. The impact of austerity is without doubt shocking and a sad reflection on one of the richest countries in the developed world. However, the above researchers and organisations make little or no reference to how these measures have impacted on BAME people's health and life chances. After years of experiencing racism in all levels of society, especially during and after the two World Wars and the rise of explicit hostile environment during the European referendum, the austerity has had a cumulative and "devastating" impact on BAME women and households Runnymede Trust (2017) (23).

The UK government's austerity measures have hit BAME people hardest, exacerbated discrimination in Britain, and further entrenched racial inequality, a United Nations report by BBC News, (2018) (24) expert has have warned, in a stinging critique of the ruling coalition government social policies. "The structural socio-economic exclusion of racial and ethnic minority communities in the United Kingdom is striking," E. Tendayi Achiume, the UN's Special rapporteur on racism and human rights said in a report. "Reliable reports have shown that the austerity measures have been disproportionately detrimental to members of racial and ethnic minority communities, who are also the hardest hit by unemployment," said Achiume, an assistant professor at UCLA School of Law. Her report came hot on the heels of a report by the UN's rapporteur on extreme poverty; Philip Alston on Sky news criticized the government's "systematic immiseration of a significant part of the British population." Reis (undated) (25) asserted that BME women have borne the brunt of cuts to benefits and gained the least from the tax cuts introduced since 2010.There is clear compounding effects of gender and racial inequalities that extends across the income distribution but is felt most acutely at the lowest incomes for Black and Asian women. Certain groups with a significant pay gap compared to white men have a smaller pay gap within their own ethnicity. For instance, the gender pay gap between Pakistani/Bangladeshi men and women is 4.9 per cent and between Black African men and women is 7.7 per cent, reflecting that both men and women in these ethnic groups are often trapped in low paid jobs and making these households the poorest on average, and most vulnerable to cuts in benefit levels that top up low wages. Britain risks following the U.S. in terms of declining life expectancy and stagnant wages for the less-educated section of the population if the causes of inequality go unchecked (McGuiness, 2019) (26). These deep measures would have significant impact on people's health and well-being, and they will end in the lap of the NHS.

Austerity and health

Austerity measures were compounded by the introduction of the Health and Social Care Act of 2012. This aimed to empower patients, by giving them a greater voice and control of their own care. It put clinicians at the centre of purchasing care, free up providers to innovate and give new focus on public health. The latter was to be transferred to the already financially challenged local authorities. Additionally, it took away the Government's ultimate responsibility to provide NHS care for all. It opened the way to changing the process for how the NHS was managed and allowed NHS trusts to contract out an increasing number of services (about 40 per cent) to private providers. Dorling (2023) (27) and Whitehead et al (2021) (28) argued that the damage caused was little noticed because the government cuts in the first round of austerity targeted local authorities and adult social care. The first group of people to see their life expectancy fall were elderly women who mostly lived on their own. It was not until 2014 that this connection became apparent. In 2015 the first 5 per cent increase in mortality was recorded and the government tried to attribute it to influenza. Austerity measures significantly impacted on and are still impacting all determinants of health. These are suitable and affordable housing, employment with inbuilt safety measures, adequate pay on sick leave, access to food, nutrition, water, affordable transport, clean air, leisure facilities, and among others support for those who are not able to work and pensions for older people who have retired. There is extremely disturbing trends that have emerged in England. Growing child poverty, homelessness and food poverty led to an unprecedented rise in infant mortality, mental health problems, and stalling life expectancy, especially for women in the poorest areas and cities. These were in areas where over ten years of austerity has hit the poorest hardest.

Stuckler et al (2017) (29) added that adults with lower income tend to have worse outcome including poorer health, lower life expectancy and lower subjective well-being than individuals with more money, although the causal links are stronger in some areas as opposed to others. Having an adequate income can reduce the risk of mental health problems such as stress, depression, and anxiety. Marmot, (2020) (30) added, "in health care terms people can expect to spend more of their lives in poor health". Improvements to life expectancy have stalled and declined for the poorest 10 per cent of women and the health gap has grown between wealthy and deprived areas. Living in a deprived area of the Northeast is worse than living in a similar deprived area in London, to the extent that life expectancy is nearly five years less. The latest finding from the Office of National Statistics (ONS) by Jones (2022) (31) revealed some alarming features. It stated life expectancy in the most deprived areas of England fell "significantly" in the three years to 2020, while the inequality gap with people living in the least deprived areas grew even wider. Jones explained that COVID-19 may be a contributing factor, but significant inequalities were obvious before the arrival of the pandemic. Both male and female life expectancy had reduced for both groups. For females it has reduced from 78.7 to 78.3 and males from 74.0 to 73.5 years.

Independent News (2018) (32) referred to a damming report from the United Nations rapporteur on poverty, condemned the UK's austerity policies as "punitive, mean-spirited and often callous"; the shock economics of austerity has been used to implement devastating new welfare policies that have hit the vulnerable hardest. The British Medical Association (BMA) (2016) (33) provided an insight into implications for health. These are reflected in an increase of the risk of winter mortality (due to the inability to afford heating) and as a range of illnesses; increased mortality among pensioners aged 85 and over, deterioration or relapse of existing health conditions, rising levels food poverty and poorer diets, increased mental health conditions, increased rates of homelessness and a notable rate of male suicide. Marmot proposed an evidence-based strategy to address the social determinants of health, the conditions in which people are born, grow, live, work and age, and which can lead to health inequalities. Research from Glasgow University and Glasgow for Population Health examined deaths in three countries over the period of 2012-2019. It found that there were 334,327 excess deaths over the expected numbers in England, Wales and Scotland. This included 237,855 excess deaths among males in England and Wales with a further 12,735 in Scotland. Among women there were 77,133 deaths recorded in England and Wales and 6564 in Scotland. The cause of these excess deaths, they state, is likely to be austerity (McLeod, 2022) (34). They do not provide any breakdown of death by ethnicity.

Austerity and its impact on the NHS

Hernandez instanced that the budgetary constraints pursued by the government for more than a decade negatively impacted on the sustainability of the NHS. It was financially protected during austerity but struggled to meet rising demand. Examples are some NHS trusts had run deficits since 2013-2014 and in 2015-2016. There is already a forecast that the NHS will overspend their allocated budgets in 2022-2023. In some cases, NHS bodies relied on temporary and unstable sources of funding to address demand. The other impact was ideological. It replicated practices from the private sector. Efficiency targets meant hospitals needed to factor in a certain amount of savings. This had implication on the waiting times in A&E departments and the growing list of patients waiting to be assessed or waiting for treatment. This currently stands at just under 8 million (November 2023) although some may be due to the lockdown and arrival of COVID-19. Furthermore, the budget allocated to the NHS was not sufficient to address the rising demand during the austerity years. This in turn affected the financial performance of NHS bodies and the quality of the health service. Institute of Public Policy Research (IPPR) think tank analysis of the NHS (2020) (35) and international data found that just before the COVID-19 crisis hit indicated:

Hospital beds - Four in five hospitals had bed occupancy levels above the acceptable safe limit (85 per cent). In three out of five hospitals, bed occupancy exceeded 90 per cent.

- **Intensive care beds** - England had just seven hundred open and unoccupied ICU beds at the end of 2019. The Southwest had access to the least, just 51.

- **Staffing** – The health service is severely understaffed, causing increased strain on healthcare professionals. For UK to meet top international standards, it would need 49,600 more long-term care workers, 70,000 more doctors, and 220,000 more nurses.

- **Innovation** – The UK is short of CT and MRI scanners compared to similar advanced countries and NHS adoption of new treatments is also markedly slower.

- **Public health** – While smoking rates were below the international average, the UK has higher levels of excess obesity and alcohol consumption.

Over and above being adversely impacted upon by austerity, BAME people had to endure even more hostility.

Austerity and "anti-immigrant" ideology

Anti- immigrant ideology is not a recent phenomenon. Finnsdottir (2019) (36) in a survey about austerity, immigration, and the far right in Central and Eastern Europe (due to freedom of movement) concluded that austerity measures have pushed certain Central and Eastern European countries into the roles of labour-sending nations. Thus, emigration and scarcity put pressure on traditional conceptions of belonging, fuelling radical politics. In this way, austerity provided the material and ideological conditions under which emigration comes to be seen as a threat to the well-being of the nation, stoking support for nationalist populist parties. This was very evident during the European Referendum. Many people from the EU were blamed for "causing social problems". Barras and Shields (2017) (37) instanced during austerity, immigrants and immigration policy have come to be a scapegoat for contributing to elevated unemployment, lowering wages, and contributing to welfare burdens and state fiscal crisis, with many calling for harsh immigrant- restricting policies (a closed borders strategy), although they point to the reality that immigration continues to be vitally important to modern societies and to neo-liberalism itself.

In the United Kingdom, much of the aforementioned information is substantiated by Simms (2016) (38). He referred to Professor Dorling of Oxford University, who claimed the fundamental reasons for worsening health and declining living standards in the UK. These are the growing economic inequality, public spending cuts and austerity. He argued immigration has been used as a scapegoat for these issues. He continued almost all other European countries tax more effectively, spend more on health, and do not tolerate our degree of economic inequality. He added the UK has been systematically underfunding education and training, increasing student loans and debt, tolerating increasingly unaffordable housing, introducing insecure work contracts and privatising the services the young will need in future. He continued that the UK has benefited from the immigration of healthier than average young adults, educated at someone else's expense; many of them work in our health, education, social, and care services, resulting in reduction in health inequalities and improved the nation's health.

The anti-immigrant ideology became much more explicit during events leading up to the European Referendum. Hirsch (2018) (39) articulated that the Labour and Conservative parties have always been eager to place limits on immigration. She continued that there has been hardening of attitudes during the 2000 to 2010 (when austerity was in full swing) and the government was upstaged by the United Kingdom Independence Party (UKIP). This continues to this day with the daily coverage by sections of the media on sending migrants to Rwanda. The latter is not seen as a radical right political party but with populist, anti-immigrant and anti-European views (Mulhall 2021) (40). UKIP has, since the 1990s, been demanding a referendum with a view to asking the British people if they wanted to stay or leave the European Union. The then Prime Minister in February 2016 finally conceded and called for a referendum. UKIP was gaining in popularity and according to Mulhall posed one of the most successful challenges to the established political parties in modern British history. What was to follow was a very traumatic time personally and for many Europeans and BAME people who have been living in Britain for decades.

UKIP launched its Eurosceptic and anti-immigrant campaign to attract the disgruntled and predominantly the disadvantaged working classes. These were the very same people who were adversely impacted by austerity measures. The political parties were critical in blaming all or most of the ills of Britain on the shoulders of all BAME and some

European people, but not austerity. BAME people who have lived here for decades were explicitly referred to as "immigrants". UKIP received 3.9 million votes at the 2015 general election, with more than a little help from various sections of the media. The Tory government panicked and made radical cuts to immigration. The campaign was exemplified by a poster with UKIP's leader in front with the headlines "at breaking point" depicting huge numbers of non-white people making their way into Europe (Mulhall and Hirsch). The poster claimed that 76 million Turkish people were coming to the UK via Europe. It was another set of events in Europe that helped to fuel the anti-immigrant sentiments. Hayden (2022) (41) instanced that in response to the arrival of asylum seekers in the EU, the latter had, since the late 1990s and early 2000s, allocated up to 2 billion Euros towards solidifying its external borders. This had two objectives: to make it much harder for asylum seekers to enter the EU and the second to appease the increasing right-wing populous. The fact that they had all signed up to the 1951 Refugee Convention was insignificant. Hayden continued and pointed out in 2015 two devastating incidents; two ships carrying asylum seekers sunk and an estimated 1,100 were thought to have perished. The dead came from many parts of the world ranging from Bangladesh to Mauritania. The arrival of hundreds of thousands of asylum seekers in Europe between 2015 and 2024 sparked a surge in anti-immigrant, xenophobic and racist sentiments across the continent. These hostilities were magnified by openly anti-immigrant views expressed in North America. These alarmed some political leaders and was capitalised on by others. The single biggest factor according to Mulhall as regards to referendum was immigration. He quoted that 90 per cent of people saw immigration as a drain on the economy and 88 per cent of those who wanted fewer immigration voted to leave the Union. It indicated that immigration had overtaken the economy as the most important deciding factor for voters.

Both Mulhall and Hirsch agreed that the working and the lower middle classes who lived in the most deprived localities and some who lived in areas with relatively low levels of immigration voted to leave the European Union. By contrast, the professional classes voted to remain. It could be argued that they were less impacted by the decade-long austerity and this may well have been a deciding factor in their decision making. Hirsch argued that there is worldwide evidence to indicate that with the rise of income inequality and the march of globalisation has corresponded remarkably to the rise of nationalism, "tribalism" and had little to do with immigration per-se. Nonetheless, immigrants continued to be blamed for among others a shortage of social housing. The main political parties were conspicuous by their absence. They failed to point out that not one of them have built adequate affordable housing when they were in government. Both were complicit in this misinformation campaign. Blame was also apportioned to immigrants abusing the NHS, welfare systems, and even causing traffic jams. It was always the case that immigration was always a topic of discussion during past general election campaigns; in 2016 Hirsch argued that it was weaponised like never before. More shocking was that some of the leave voters were themselves "immigrants" or descendent of "immigrants".

The referendum campaign impacted on me in several ways. It affected my mental health to the point that I did not want to listen to the news or listen to the grossly inaccurate and racist way in which all immigrants were tarnished. It seemed to go on for eternity. There was no end of micro-aggression by way of non-verbal communication and uncomfortable glances and eye contact which indicated vile hostility from many, exclusively white people. Before the EU referendum the hostilities were always there but it was not so overt. Now it was in my face and done with impunity. Many incidents took place during this time but two stand out: I called a company to do some work at my house. An operative arrived and we discussed the work and suddenly he asked me "what brings you here?" I certainly did not expect this and was stunned. I replied, "I am retired from the NHS". A stranger came into my property and asked me that question? Would the operative ask a white person the same question in the same context? The other was a charity I supported used to send a man to collect my donation monthly. He had been doing so for a year. On that day, he arrived and from my front door he saw a picture, a map of Egypt and asked me if I was from there. I replied "no". He retorted "what are you doing here then?" And very quickly took off. I had no opportunity reply. I never saw him again. I have no doubt that these incidents were related to the vile anti-immigrant ambiance that was and is still prevailing. Hirsch outlined there was a 40 per cent increase in racially and religiously aggravated crime during the months after the results of the referendum was announced. 17.4 million people in Britain voted to leave the European Union. These were also directed to the members of the Polish and other European communities, and one person was killed when he was heard speaking in the Polish language. The referendum campaign exploited people's fears. Facts were not seen as relevant; it was perception that mattered (Hirsch).

The hostile environment policy was designed to make Britain a very hostile place for illegal immigrants. Most of the populous are not able to distinguish between legal and illegal migrants, so we are all lumped in one group. This started in 2013 by the former Labour government and continued by the Home Secretary Mrs Theresa May from 2010-2016. Mrs May took the hostile environment to a different level and made a pledge to reduce immigration to the "tens of thousands". The Windrush scandal was a central part of that objective. Gentleman (2022) (42) argued that the Windrush Scandal was 29 years in the making in a report of a Home Office commissioned paper which officials have repeatedly tried to suppress. The 52-page report analysed by an unnamed historian argued how the British Empire depended on a racist ideology to function. In continued, during the period 1950-1981 every single piece of immigration or citizenship legislation was designed at least in part to reduce the number of people with black or brown skin who were permitted to live and work in the UK. The scandal itself reared its head in 2013 but came to a crescendo in April 2018. It saw hundreds of British Caribbean citizens who have been living and working in the UK since 1945 wrongly targeted by immigration enforcement officers because of the government's Hostile Environment Policy and changes to the Immigration laws. Consequently, specifically black British-Caribbean British people were suddenly barred from working; refused access to government services, lost access to their bank accounts, pensions, welfare benefits and access the NHS care. In certain instances, Joint Council for Welfare of Immigrants (JCWI 2020) (43) stated that individuals were detained and deported. The arrival of COVID-19 saw East Asians were also facing the brunt of what is called "hate crime". There were frequent reports that Chinese and East Asian people were experiencing a rise in physical and verbal attacks. Many were abused simply for "looking like Chinese" or East Asians and some were physically attacked (Grey and Hansen 2021) (43).

On the political front, after the shock result of the European referendum election, the then Prime Minister David Cameron swiftly resigned and Mrs Theresa May (who oversaw the Windrush scandal as Home Secretary) was elected as the second female Prime Minister on 13 July 2016. After about three years her tenure at Number 10 Downing Street was over. She was replaced by Boris Johnson who was elected in December 2019 as Prime Minister after one of the most unpredictable general elections. He won with an eighty-two-seat majority. His agenda was to "Get Brexit Done". With this healthy majority, Boris Johnson was able to go full steam ahead to get the

"Brexit divorce" deal through the House of Parliament. This was completed on 31 January 2020. Little did he know that he was to face his biggest challenge; COVID-19 arrived in January 2020.

Conclusion

This chapter has discussed the antecedent to the over a decade long austerity measures. These measures were implemented despite national and international objections. Instead the coalition government proceeded with drastic financial cuts in almost every institution. The decade long austerity has had an indelible impact on the life chances of many people. This impacted disproportionately on the most deprived communities and people in these communities. Older people were the hardest hit, as well as those who lived in deprived areas. These measures impacted on people's physical and mental health, and reduced life expectancy with more people living with increasing morbidity. BAME people were disproportionately impacted upon. Some politicians and sections of the media were instrumental in using the effects of austerity and turned into 'anti-immigrant' sentiments, exacerbating the already hostile environment. Unfortunately, it was used and exploited by some politicians to whip up 'anti-immigrant' feelings and all these contributed to further ill-health and reduced life chances of particularly BAME people. There is a strong body of evidence to suggest BAME people have for decades been poorly served by society and the NHS. All the evidence discussed above indicates austerity had and is still having a detrimental impact on the social determinants of health.

In the first part of this journey, we have taken a route from my birthplace where I experienced racism without knowing it and the start of my journey in the NHS. I outlined the birth of the latter and the ideological and political values which underpinned it. We explored how BAME staff and patients were and are still being treated. This is supplemented by an overview of Race Relations after two World Wars, the contribution of BAME soldiers in these wars and the presence of BAME people in Britain. We then discussed more recent development like austerity and its deep impact on life chances. In part 2 we explore how racism was brutally exposed again when COVID-19 arrived.

Part Two
BRITAIN AND COVID-19

CHAPTER 8
BRITAIN'S STATE OF READINESS FOR COVID-19

This chapter discusses the extent to which Britain, and England in particular, was prepared for the arrival of COVID-19[11] (also called coronavirus). England's state of readiness is placed in the context of race relations, racism in the wider society, the NHS, and fourteen years of austerity. They all have significant implications on the social determinants of health, particularly for BAME people. After being blamed for the ills of Britain, feeling the impact of Islamophobia, austerity measures and among others the Windrush scandal, now we are faced with a deadly virus.

For some years Britain has had policies and procedures in place to respond to outbreaks of new infections by having institutional arrangements to facilitate effective action. As part of this an exercise named Cygnus was carried out in 2016 by the government (Pegg, 2020) (1). It was a three-day simulation of a flu outbreak to assess the UK's readiness to respond to a

---

[11] In January 2020, the World Health Organisation (WHO) informed the world that a cluster of cases of pneumonia of unknown cause was detected in Wuhan City (China). On the 12th of January, the virus was identified as COVID-19. Coronavirus disease also known as COVID-19 is an infectious disease caused by a newly discovered virus. Most people infected with the COVID-19 virus would experience mild to moderate respiratory symptoms and recover without requiring special treatment. Older people and those with underlying medical problems like cardiovascular disease, diabetes, chronic respiratory disease, and cancer are more likely to be impacted. COVID-19 spreads primarily through droplets of saliva or discharge from the nose when an infected person coughs or sneezes. This was to cause a global pandemic.

pandemic. 950 officials from central and local government, NHS organisations, prisons, and local emergency response planners participated. The simulation asked participants to imagine they were fighting a fictitious "worst-case-scenario" flu pandemic affecting up to 50 per cent of the population and causing up to 400,000 excess deaths. Over the three days all were told to imagine they were managing the seventh week of the pandemic which placed a very high demand on health and social care. The simulation was not only to test how emergency services would respond but also to present to ministers and officials the type of environment within which they would be making decisions. A report was compiled the following year and distributed among participants. The findings were,

"The UK's preparedness and response, in terms of its plans, policies and capability, was currently not sufficient to cope with the extreme demands of a severe pandemic that would have a nationwide impact across all sectors".

Although different government departments had their own plans, which enabled a flexible response, no one had oversight of the entire plan. This would result in much difficulty in shifting resources between departments and to respond to unpredictable needs. Pegg quoted from the report:

"The lack of joint tactical level plans was evidenced when the scenario demand for services outstripped the capacity of local responders, in the areas of excess deaths, social care and the NHS".

It was very difficult to locate beds in care homes as they were almost all privately run. In addition, problematic issues were highlighted as regards to providing the levels of support needed, if it became necessary to move patients into the care home sector. The latter was already working under significant pressure. This could well be exacerbated in the event of the pandemic with staff going off sick and widespread infection spreading in care homes. The report made 22 recommendations to government. It suggested that further work was needed to understand the capacity of the care sector and how the public would react to the crisis. It identified the creation of a 'joint-level tactical plan' to help different organisations cooperate more effectively. The simulation report was not widely published and there are questions whether the recommendations were taken in full.

According to Ary News (2020) (2) Professor Sridhar of Global Public Health warned in 2018 how a corona virus type outbreak would arrive in Britain. Professor Sridhar, a prominent leader in global public health at Edinburgh University, predicted with uncanny accuracy how the next major threat to UK health would evolve. Someone in China would become infected by an animal. They would get on a plane to Britain and infect others. She challenged as to why Britain was worried about what was happening here.

"It's about interconnections across the world. If you want to solve these problems, you can't do it on a go alone approach".

This was not the first virus to emerge from that kind of setting. The lessons from the 2013 Ebola outbreak have transformed the responses of both World Health Organisation (WHO) and scientists. They previously competed for results but are now pooling resources together to an unprecedented degree. The WHO sent officers to China and concluded that (1) the virus was extremely dangerous and (2) China had resorted to the most aggressive disease containment effort in history, i.e. hand washing, mask-wearing, all government and all society-wide approach. This included clearing giant hospitals to make way for virus hit patients and imposing drastic restrictions on movement. According to Shipman (2020) (3) another structural deficit was that Britain had no major outbreak epicentre. This was compounded by "big rift between health establishment and politicians".

When COVID-19 struck, the UK government did not learn lessons from previous pandemics in parts of Asia and particularly South Korea. They developed extra beds for hospital isolation and rooms were equipped with facilities for renal dialysis and ventilation capacity (to help patients breathe mechanically). By early January 2020 they were already detecting cases and responding to outbreaks that were occurring. Professor Devi Sridhar related places like West Africa, deployed their past Ebola structures towards managing COVID-19. Poorer nations are all too aware of the destruction infectious diseases can cause. Consequently, they tend to react much faster. It is conceivable that the complacency may have been due to the declaration by John Hopkins Global Health Security Index (the most comprehensive global study into pandemic preparedness) that Britain was the second best prepared in the world after USA. There was another factor that preoccupied the government: Brexit.

In 2016 Britain voted to leave the European Union and the wave of elation and hysteria was still very palpable. There was an even stronger flavour of nationalism, populism, and a sense of Britain was to rule the waves. The political class were not keen to listen and learn of what good practice was emerging from other countries. A colonial undertone cannot be ruled out. The government's focus was to protect the NHS from being overwhelmed and was not receptive to emerging international best practice. Requests for instituting testing were not heeded. The World Health Organisation warned on 24th February 2020 that the extremely dangerous virus was on its way and recommended "Test, Test and Test". However, there was little action. There should have been a society-wide approach consisting of handwashing, mask wearing, imposing restrictions on movement of people, and making room for patients in hospitals. The availability of ventilators, teams of test and tracing were not acted upon, and the lockdown should have been implemented much sooner.

BMJ (2020) (4) referred to the simulation exercise and provided a much wider contextual analysis of the response to COVID-19. It argued that the UK response so far had been neither well-prepared nor remotely adequate. This was supported by Hopkins (2020) (5) who added that when it did respond, the government's plan was lethargic, confusing and geared towards herd immunity (allowing most people to be infected with the virus). Hopkins quoted a statement made by the Prime Minister, "what is happening in other countries doesn't necessarily mirror what is happening in the UK". This typified the go-it -alone mentality that took hold in the government circles. Hopkins noted that the Prime Minister did not attend five COBRA (Cabinet Office Briefing Room A) meetings with European leaders to discuss the need for medical equipment. It warned of high levels of need for mechanical ventilation and high death rates. These warnings were ignored by the UK government (BMJ). Italy went into full lockdown by 11th March, closely followed by Spain and France while Britain rejected lockdown on the belief that the population would not accept it. As the death toll began to rise, the Prime Minister was catapulted into action. A strict lockdown[12] was announced on 23rd March 2020 and it was implemented the next day. BMJ questioned as to why the government announced a move from the containment to the delay phase. NHS 111 and Public Health teams working on contact tracing were confused and overwhelmed. Instead of following the WHO's standard containment approach to find, test, treat and isolate which worked well in other countries testing and tracing was stopped. BMJ and Hopkins are very critical of the constitution of the SAGE (Scientific Advisory Group for

---

[12] This was embodied by three words. STAY HOME, PROTECT THE NHS, SAVE LIVES. Essentially we were to work from home if possible, not to mix with people outside our household, to access shops for essentials, have limited access to health care, shops, restaurants, pubs, cafes were to close. Police were to monitor these restrictions.

Emergencies) none of the three members were experts in developing and implementing public health response. BMJ is particularly scathing about the discharging of older patients to care homes without testing if they had COVID-19. It called this policy "reckless". By the time the lockdown was announced there was a consensus that almost two months of potential preparation and prevention had been squandered.

Taylor (2022) (6) pointed before the pandemic arrived there were around 100,000 NHS staff vacancies and some rundown buildings. Jeremy Hunt, the previous Secretary of State for Health from 2012-2018, concurred and admitted he was "too slow to boost the NHS workforce". The NHS has had significant workforce challenges for decades. To compensate for staff shortage, Shipman et al (2020) (7) suggested the NHS resorted to allocating health care assistants into intensive care units. Untrained staff were given minimal training to monitor complex life-saving machinery, such as ventilators. Staff who were mobilised were from out-patients departments, operating theatres, and general nursing departments. Deals were struck with private hospitals for availability of beds, more ventilators, 10,000 nurses, 700 doctors and 8000 clinical staff.

PPE availability and suitability

The lack of preparedness cascaded from the government all the way to the clinical staff and this was more acutely reflected in the availability, provision and suitability of Personal Protective Equipment (PPE)[13]. In terms of availability of PPE my own daily records (gathered during the Daily Briefings by Downing Street) indicated that there were significant problems with the availability of PPE at least during the middle of April 2020. This is supported by the media and Hoernke et al (2021) (8) who

---

[13] PPE is equipment that protects the wearer against health and safety risks at work. It ranges from basic items such as masks, aprons, gowns, and disposable gloves to specialised items, like face shields and respirator masks. Some workers also wear medical devices such as surgical masks to protect patients against infection

reported that stockpiles were running low from the beginning of March 2020 across the country. Visors, full length fluid repellent gowns, and fluid repellent masks were especially in short supply. At the start of the pandemic the advice from Public Health England was that staff who encountered COVID-19 patients while not wearing PPE should continue to work unless they developed symptoms. This advice was removed later. The National Audit Office (NAO) (2020) (9) supported the broad thrust of the research by Hoernke. It added "there are important aspects that could and should have been done much better in supplying PPE". The government recognised very early on that demand was quickly outstripping supply, but it took a long time for it to receive the large volumes of PPE ordered, particularly from new suppliers which created significant risks (more on PPE in the next chapter).

Much emphasis was placed on the local Public Health departments. Lee et al (2020) (10) and the BMJ argued that during the austerity years there had been significant disinvestment in Public Health. Its operational budget has been cut by up to 40 per cent between 2013 and 2019. The other change was that Public Health departments were transferred from the NHS to the already financially challenged Local Authorities. These would have implications for workforce stability and potential loss of expertise. Lee et al continued both Public Health England (PHE) and the wider health system were not adequately prepared for the possible pandemic threats. PHE, they argued, lacked the information technology infrastructure to deal with large scale pandemics. In addition, any emergency planning carried out was focused not on the pandemic threats but on the potential consequences of Brexit.

Oborne (2021) (11) suggested that John Hopkins University published a study on countries who were the best prepared to handle the pandemic. It concluded that the United States was judged to be the most prepared and Britain, the second. The reality was Britain had the second highest death rate in Western Europe. The number of deaths on 7 May 2024 was 232,112. The COVID-19 tracker has been stopped as of 13 April 2024. The government had to choose between inflicting damage to the economy or saving lives. Furthermore, the state of readiness of Britain to meet the virus head on did not factor in the political leadership. The Prime Minister appeared on various TV channels with the mantra "as far as possible it should be business as usual for the overwhelming majority of this country". He claimed to be shaking hands with everybody (Wood, 2020) (12). The virus stopped him in his tracks. He contracted the virus and was hospitalised. In accordance with the business-as-usual mantra in mid-March, the sporting authorities allowed the Cheltenham Festival with crowds of around 150,000 to go ahead, and a week earlier the Prime Minister attended the Six Nations rugby match at Twickenham. Another sporting event that went ahead was the European Champions league football match between Liverpool and Atletico Madrid in Liverpool. It had an attendance of 54,000 spectators. These events turned out to be super spreaders (Conn, 2020) (13). Oborne concluded that the government was slow to stop public events. It ditched the test and trace strategy early only to return to it later, wasted time with a dangerous (herd) immunity strategy, and missed the deadline for a joint EU (European Union) ventilator procurement scheme. It also failed to introduce its test and trace application on time. In March 2020, Gregory of Sunday Times highlighted the acute shortages of medicines as demands surged for painkillers, anti-depressants, anti-anxiety, and anti-inflammatory medication. Tucker et al (2020) (14) also of Sunday Times reflected on the fact that thousands of passengers from coronavirus hotspots such as Iran, Italy, and even China were flying to the UK despite the government lockdown. The European block banned virtually all travellers from outside for thirty days. They quoted a government spokesperson who claimed there is "no evidence that closing borders or travel bans would have any effect on the spread of infection". Critics would assert that these arguments have been made with the benefit of hindsight. However, there was ample advice provided by the WHO, emerging good practice from some European countries and South Asian countries. There was a group think mentality of going it alone and many missed opportunities to participate in Europe wide strategies. The Test and Trace strategy that was repeatedly advised by WHO was stopped in early March 2020. Ports and borders were also left fully operational. There is unambiguous evidence that the advice from the simulation exercise were not fully taken on board. In the final analysis according to Professor Sridhar, this crisis was entirely preventable.

COVID-19 is here

COVID-19 found Britain (in this case England) in a poor state of readiness. The first reported cases of the virus in the United Kingdom were identified in late January 2020. By 23rd March, when a national lockdown prohibiting non-essential movement was announced, reported cases had increased to over 6,000. However, these were probably a small fraction of total infections because most COVID-19 cases were mild or even asymptomatic (Jit et al, 2020) (15). Death rates (ONS 2021) (16) were 3,912 involving coronavirus that occurred in March 2020 in England and Wales; of these, 3,372 (86 per cent) had COVID-19 assigned as the underlying cause of death. This propelled the government to announce a lockdown on 24 March 2020. Sparrow et al (2020) (17) pointed out the lockdown stipulated that people were to stay at home, police would be called to enforce this directive, businesses were ordered to close, those who were able to work from home should do so. Individuals could only go outdoor for exercise and to shop for essentials, social distancing of two metres was enforced, and attendance for medical appointments for the extremely vulnerable. The mantra was "Stay Home, Protect the NHS, Save Lives". The emphasis was on "Protect the NHS" code for preventing the NHS to be "overwhelmed".

From National Health Service to National COVID-19 Service

On the 17th March 2020, NHS Chief Executive Sir Simon Stevens, and Chief Operating Officer Amanda Pritchard published its detailed action plan (NHSE) (18). Briefly, the actions were, to free up hospital beds by discharging patients who were "medically fit", maximise the availability of staff by closing departments, postpone planned operations and "stress test operation readiness". This meant freeing up to 30,000 beds and make maximum use of the independent sector. Other requirements were to ensure oxygen supply and distribution was in working order. The NHS should purchase additional mechanical ventilators and ensure the availability of PPE. Refresher training should be provided for staff and patients with respiratory problems should be segregated. Mental health, learning disability and autism providers needed to make plans for COVID-19 patients. Staff who relinquished their registration could return to work and other staff to work beyond their usual field of expertise. GPs needed to support older and vulnerable patients, roll out remote consultation using available technology, and provide enhanced support for those in need. For service users, there was much reduced access to primary care and other preventative aspects of health would without doubt lead to more serious illness further down the line. This would result in increased morbidity and mortality. Effectively, it meant that the NHS stopped providing services it was designed for. In layperson terms during that period, it was feasible to die from cancer, strokes, health attacks, and any other illnesses but NOT from COVID-19. All the focus was on

COVID-19. As Smyth (2022) (19) stated, thousands of middle-aged people were dying of heart conditions because they did not get statins or blood pressure medicines during the pandemic. The Chief Medical Officer Professor Chris Whitty warned that a higher numbers of deaths than normal were probably due to preventable conditions.

Conclusion

This chapter has discussed when COVID-19 was on its way, it found the government asleep at the wheels. Lessons from the simulation exercise were not learnt nor were lessons that were emerging from other countries. The Prime Minister wanted "to carry on as normal" until he was infected by the virus. Some major sporting events were held with thousands of people in attendance, and they are or were called 'super spreaders'. All airports and arrival by sea carried on as normal. Both these sporting events and the open entry added to a rise of infections and consequently a high number of deaths. Eventually, the government was forced to act and the NHS stopped functioning as normal. It became a National COVID-19 Service in March 2020. The entire focus was to Stay Home, Protect the NHS, Save Lives. In the words of Professor Sridhar this crisis was entirely preventable. The then Prime Minister missed some meetings to discuss the supply of PPE and ventilators. The lack of national state of readiness cascaded all the way to the front line staff. This was manifested in the availability, accessibility, and suitability of PPEs. These were lacking at the very outset of the pandemic and continued to be the case, at least during the first wave. Many departments were closed or provided limited services. Many staff were relocated to areas with COVID-19 patients. Health care assistants were given basic training to monitor very challenging medical cases. Staff who were in training were allowed to practice and those who had relinquished their registration were permitted to return to practice often not in their field of expertise.

There is no dispute that many front line workers were left at an increased risk of getting infected. Access to primary care was very limited. Most consultations were conducted by phone and face to face interactions were at a premium. There was a distinct view that the government was torn between saving lives and saving the economy. The planning or lack of Brexit was also a factor in the poor preparation for the arrival of COVID-19. Essentially, it was reasonable to die from any other diseases but not from coronavirus. Nonetheless, Britain had the highest death rate from COVID-19 in Western Europe. Many in the medical profession were significantly worried that the delay in getting early care would have a boomerang effect. Given this context how did the poor state of readiness and PPE shortage impact on particularly NHS staff?

CHAPTER 9
COVID-19 AND BAME STAFF IN THE NHS

In chapter two there was extensive discussion about the treatment of BAME doctors and nurses in the NHS before COVID-19 struck. Many faced and are still facing discrimination even before they start their careers in the NHS. This chapter discusses the experience of NHS BAME doctors and nurses when COVID- 19 arrived. It is framed within the context of British colonial exploits, the notion of white superiority, racist events, the European Referendum, and among others the Windrush scandal.

As the virus raged across Britain, a significant number of BAME doctors and nurses were dying at an alarming rate. Media commentators during the early phase of COVID-19 suggested an over-representation of BAME staff, especially in mortality rates. Chaudhry et al (2020) (1) highlighted that of 1.2 million staff employed by the NHS, 20.7 per cent belong to BAME ethnicity. During the initial phase, analysis of NHS staff deaths showed that 64 percent of those who died were of BAME ethnicity. Cook et al (22/4/2020) (2) using three investigators collected data separately and examined various forms of evidence based on staff ethnicity, the departments they worked at, and in what capacity. In most cases ethnicity was identified by pictures of individuals. Many were of BAME ethnicity, born outside the UK, and among Caucasians a number was born in Europe. Overall, these doctors tended to be older than other staff members and the vast majority were male.

The main findings indicated that 64 per cent of nurses and 95 per cent of doctors died from COVID-19, while only around 17 per cent of the UK population were of BAME ethnicity. The absence of certain workforce groups among those who died is noted. More BAME individuals died compared to their proportion in the overall population. It was not possible to ascertain where they contracted the infection, whether at home or at work, but most individuals who died had both patient-facing roles and were actively working during the pandemic. It seemed highly likely that many would have contracted coronavirus during work. The higher number of deaths among Filipino staff (mainly nurses) has also been highlighted by Ikharia (2020) (3). At that time there was an estimated 20,000 Filipino staff employed in the NHS and constituted a significant proportion of the nursing workforce. The Filipino Nurses Association estimated that 20 per cent of its nurse members died during the pandemic. On some occasions a doctor stood outside a hospital with a poster "Protect NHS care workers" which was to draw attention to the fate of NHS staff who were working on the front line. Bhatia (2020) (4) after referring to further research concluded that over 50 per cent of all deaths reported within the NHS were from health workers born outside the UK (this is identifiable as death certificates require the recording place of birth and not ethnicity). This represented less than 18 per cent of the NHS health workforce. The first eleven deaths reported were among doctors working in the NHS who were all BAME ethnicity. In May 2020 an analysis in the Guardian by Marsh and McIntyre (2020) (5) concurred. The number of healthcare workers who died from COVID-19 has reached 200 and more than 6 in 10 of the victims were of BAME ethnicity. Staff in other hospitals in mental health, GP surgeries, care homes and other settings found that 122 of the deceased or 61 per cent of the total were of BAME ethnicity. Of those staff whose ethnicity could be identified, Asian workers accounted for 34 per cent of the overall death toll, Black staff 24 per-cent (making a total of 58 per-cent. White workers were 36 per cent, and the rest were unknown. In September of 2020 the British Medical Association (BMA) (2020) (6) held a memorial in memory of the 47 doctors who died while working during the early phase of the pandemic. The BMA council chair said

"They are GPs and hospital doctors who treat us when we are sick and they are our friends and colleagues, who dedicated their lives in the pursuit of helping us get better. The vast majority who have sadly died are of BAME ethnicity, with many coming from overseas to contribute their valuable skills and expertise to the NHS to save lives of others only to tragically lose their own. He added we must never allow our BAME colleagues to be taken for granted or disadvantaged".

The numbers of BAME staff dying varied during different periods of the pandemic, but there is no doubt that BAME staff were significantly over-represented in mortality figures. The causes were associated with problems with the availability of suitable and appropriate PPE, increased exposure to the virus, lack of comprehensive risk assessments followed by management and the working conditions they were exposed to. It has been well- established that most of BAME staff operate in front line roles.

Availability of Personal Protective Equipment (PPE)
At the very outset the availability of appropriate and suitable PPE emerged as a significant concern. My notes from the daily briefings of the lockdown throughout the duration of the pandemic indicated that from the start of the lockdown (24 March 2020) there were consistent reports of major problems in the availability of PPE. This was confirmed

by the COVID-19 government's procurement and supply of PPE (UK Parliament) (2021) (7). Front line workers were left

"Risking their lives to provide treatment and care and PPE shortages affected frontline workers especially during the first wave for those operating in health and social care sector".

Some staff purchased their own PPE from DIY stores as face masks provided were of limited use and was not reaching the right places. Availability of PPE was beset by distribution problems to running out of masks and gowns. At least one NHS trust decided to fly in PPE from China. Hoernke et al (2021) (8) conducted forty-six semi-structured in-depth telephone interviews with front line workers, examined media and social media posts and examined twenty-five PPE policies. Health Care Workers (HCWs) using social media expressed concerns that PPE stockpiles were running low from the start of March 2020 across the country. Visors, full length fluid repellent gowns and masks were especially in short supply. PHE guidance stated that respirators needed to be the correct size, fit tested before use and that HCWs were not to proceed if a "good fit" could not be achieved. Many reported that the respirators failed the fit test. A lack of alternatives meant that practitioners proceeded caring for patients with COVID-19 with them or used equipment that provided a lower level of protection. Other concerns highlighted the suitability of PPE for BAME HCWs. PPE specification failed to consider that staff may be wearing turbans, sporting beards or head scarves. There was a strong impression that the face masks and other facial equipment were designed on the model of a 'white face'. Other media reported that primary care received shipments of PPE, but they were years out of date. The National Health Service England, (NHSE) on the other hand stipulated that these were tested, had passed stringent tests, and demonstrated that they were safe.

HCWs found creative ways to limit the use of PPE. They attended fewer ward rounds (where patient care would be reviewed by several HCWs) and did not enter certain areas. Just before the lockdown the DHSC announced that there were local distribution problems although they had adequate national supply. Other reports argued that there were enough PPE to go round but they were a precious resource and needed to be used where there was clinical need. Hoernke et al concluded that at the start of the pandemic HCWs' reported limited PPE guidance leading them to care for patients suspected of suffering from COVID-19 without appropriate PPE. There was inconsistent and confusing guidance which changed frequently. In early 2020 these changed daily. Consequently, this led to confusion, distrust, and a lack of confidence in the messaging. As the pandemic became rampant some HCWs felt overwhelmed by the increasing amount of guidance from multiple sources. HCWs in the most critical areas such as critical care, emergency and respiratory departments reported inadequate training of how to safely don PPE while others identified training gaps. Although some had training in the management of flu, this was not compatible with COVID-19 requirements. There was a strong view that HCWs interviewed stated the lack of "if we are not protected, we can't protect the public".

Lack of PPE increased their exposure to COVID-19. This particularly applied to HCWs who had underlying health conditions or were BAME men, pregnant women or those who have been redeployed. The front line workers operating in critical care, emergency and respiratory departments were redeployed from primary, secondary, and tertiary care across the UK. Furthermore, changing facility shortages meant that staff wore potentially contaminated clothes home and exposed their family members to the virus. At the early stages of the pandemic PHE advised HCWs who encountered COVID-19 patients while not wearing PPE should remain at work unless they developed symptoms. This guidance was later removed. Harewood (2021) (9) added that Health Care Assistants worked with flimsy equipment which were not fit for purpose. This also coincided with the 'strong black' man stereotypes, meaning black men are strong and therefore would be more resistant from catching the virus.

Both the National Audit Office (NOA) (2020) (10) and UK Parliament Committees (2021) (11) argued that the government believed that it was well placed to manage the COVID-19 pandemic because it had a plan and a stockpile of PPE. The latter were designed for influenza pandemic and the plans, stockpile and PPE distribution arrangements were inadequate for the coronavirus. This was compounded when the demand for PPE rose exponentially and overwhelmed the government. This led to 'parallel supply chain' to purchase and distribute PPE. According to the NAO it took a long time to receive the large volumes of PPE, particularly from the new suppliers and thus created significant risks. There were also further difficulties with distribution to providers and many front line workers reported experiencing shortages of PPE as a result. Another shortcoming was that social care providers felt unsupported. The government failed to be transparent about decisions, publish contracts in a timely manner or maintain proper records of key decisions. It left the state open to accusations of poor value for money, conflicts of interest and preferential treatment to some suppliers. This led to undermining trust in government procurement that the Department of Health and Social Care (DHSC) has spent over £12 billion on PPE. Both ONS and www.parliament.uk noted that items worth hundreds of millions of pounds of PPE were unusable for their intended purposes, putting the efficient use of taxpayers' money at further risk. Pogrund and Glover (2022) (12) after their investigation uncovered that a total of £4.4 billion were spent by the government to purchase PPE from six companies of which £615 million worth were unused. One company received £7.4 billion in contracts but also produced more than £1 billion in PPE placed in the *"do not supply lane"* as of June 2021. These meant masks, gowns and gloves in question had not been sent to NHS staff or patients for front line use. In total more than 680 firms, including listed firms and those run by overseas contracts were to supply PPE to the UK government. In September 2021 a health minister disclosed that as of 10 June 2021 there had been £1.9 billion of stock marked *"Do not supply"*. This meant for reasons including, but not limited to, they were not *"fit for use"* because they did not pass safety tests or if they did, the PPE had passed their sell by date. An exclusive report (14/1/2023) by Siddle and White (2023) (13) of The Mirror revealed that a company paid £11 million to deliver PPE and would be paid £4.5 million to incinerate it. It is not clear if these were the PPE that the firm has produced but it confirmed that these PPEs were not fit for purpose.

Oliver (2021) (14) argued the failure to provide PPE to health and social care services has highlighted the disintegration of any culture of integrity, transparency, honesty and support for health care staff from the government and NHS providers. He was shown a database of over 1500 anonymised stories from their nationally available app. They described trusts failing to supply doctors with PPE that met the official specifications stipulated by Public Health England or failed to meet the respondents' own expectations of quality, safety and availability. The associations also listed over 200 cases of staff being threatened, bullied, unsupported, silenced or warned for speaking up over PPE use in their organisations. Oliver submitted a number of requests under the Freedom of Information Act to the NHS but did not receive answers. He pointed out that the responses he received were miles from "the open learning culture" that the DHSC and NHSE officially embraced, or the duty of candour, transparency, and openness required of doctors and nurses. In a conference proceeding held by Health and Race Observatory (15) in May 2021 Dr Chaand Nagpaul stated that during the first phase of COVID-19, 85 per cent of doctors who died were from ethnic minority backgrounds and the majority were International Medical Graduates (IMG). A BMA tracker survey found that ethnic minority doctors were twice as likely to have felt pressured to see patients with COVID-19 without adequate PPE. BAME doctors were three times as likely to have reported feeling afraid to speak up about safety issues due to fear of recrimination and/or adversely affecting their career progression. BAME doctors were less likely to report that appropriate adjustments had been made following their risk assessments and they were more likely to fail PPE fit testing. They were primarily designed to fit faces with no beards, the wearing of a turban or any other form of head covering. During a discussion there were anecdotes that in some cases hospital managers hid PPEs. ITN news (16) completed the biggest survey of its kind on 13 May 2020. It used data from 2000 HCWs focussing on the number of deaths of BAME NHS staff. Many of whom have lost colleagues from COVID-19. Respondents made the following statements:

"They don't care about us".

"Will be leaving the NHS after this".

"There is a fear of going off sick and being judged or a view that you are bringing infection in the hospital".

"Disproportionately allocated to COVID-19 wards".

Told *"to keep quiet and carry on".*

"We don't feel it in our hearts to say no, or stop going on to wards may be judged as seen as 'can't cope' even if we have issues with PPE",

Filipino nurse. 84 per cent BAME staff stated they were deployed on front line, high-risk areas and high-risk of exposure to the virus, while white staff were given time off. 73 per cent pointed to a lack of PPE and there was a fear of losing your job if they spoke out or complained. Other comments were:

"It feels as if we have been assigned to the role of foot soldiers without adequate support or protection".

There is a lack of representation at senior management and consequently many do not feel heard and BAME

"Staff death will be brushed off without much changes or protection".

Ramamurthy et al (2022) (17) research identified some specific issues which affected BAME nurses. Most are allocated night duty which is the most unpopular shift. This has been occurring for decades, and I witnessed that in the 1970s and 1980s. There is much evidence since the 1970s, that the chance of promotion is very limited. As a result, many BAME nurses opt for the night shift simply to "get out of the way and the politics". It was a way of surviving the system. The availability of PPE was a significant concern. Some PPE would run out at night, but nurses could not access new ones as in some units they were locked. Other grounds for refusing PPE were "it would scare patients". Some nurses therefore brought their own PPE to keep them safe. A BAME agency nurse challenged a procedure and was removed from her role of allocating PPE and had her contract terminated. The latest information according to the BBC, Burns (2024) (18) is that nearly 70 staff are taking their case to the High Court to sue the NHS and other employers for compensation. They allege that they caught the virus while at work and were not provided with adequate PPE.

Risk Assessment

Risk assessments are part of the management of risks in the workplace, enabling employers to decide upon reasonable steps to protect their staff and ultimately patients. It allows employers to fulfil their legal duty of care to protect their staff from harm, injury, or illness. It is important to consider and support all staff in organisations and carry out suitable and sufficient risk assessments, where there is a risk to the health, safety, and welfare of employees. Risk assessment is an on-going process and needs to be followed by actions to mitigate and reduce risk to patients, visitors and staff. As COVID-19 arrived, NHSE required health trusts in June 2020 to undertake full scale risk assessments. COVID-19 affected those who were more vulnerable to serious illness and death. Risk scoring and individual risk assessments would help employers to assess the level of risk to their workforce. To this end, the NHS Employers and NHSE provided additional guidance. This included a risk assessment of the environment itself, the workforce and the individuals that were allocated to these departments. These included, identification of the hazards, who might be harmed and how, what was being done to control the crisis, what further action was needed to control the risks, who needed to carry out this action and by when.

Khunti et al (2020) (19) from Health Education England recommended the assessment should be completed by a line manager, supervisor, designated senior manager or health and safety representative. This had to be on a one-to-one consultation with their staff in a sensitive manner and taking into consideration staff mental well-being. Employers needed to ensure that cultural factors are also taken into consideration so that staff have confidence to openly discuss and resolve their concerns. These needed to include age, sex, underlying health conditions, ethnicity, pregnancy and disability. The risk assessment for women who were 28 weeks pregnant was later changed. It stated that the risk assessment needed to focus on individual cases and not solely on pregnancy. These would no doubt have implications for pregnant staff themselves and for those who did the assessment. All risk assessments need to result in risk management.

Jesuthasan et al (2021) (20) revealed that many participants felt risk assessments had not been treated seriously by their managers and organisations. Some felt their employer organisations accommodated their identified increased risks, but many reported not seeing tangible protective actions for vulnerable ethnic minority staff. By not emphasising the importance of completing risk assessments and taking minimal action, management made staff feel the assessment was a tick box exercise. It was not seen as a strategy to reduce staff risk. A doctor described the process and its implication for her. The assessment fitted on a side of A5, she scored high, and it was recommended that she limits patient contact. However, the onus was on her to do the "chasing" and it took a few weeks to get a move off patient–facing work. The BMA chairman in the same article by BBC News, stated that it appeared white doctors found it easier to avoid patient-facing work. In a conference proceeding in May 2021, Dr Nagpaul argued that BAME doctors were less likely to report that appropriate adjustments had been made following their assessment. Ramamurthy et al concurred. BAME nurses stated that they did not get timely risk assessments despite having some severe underlying health conditions, and some got infected which could have been avoidable. White nurses appeared to be able to get shielding letters far easier than BAME nurses. The latter group were still sent to high-risk areas even when they had underlying conditions. The only senior BAME nurse was excluded from risk assessment meeting. There were reports that BAME nurses were refused swab tests while white nurses from the same trust received them.

Exacerbation of bullying and racism

It has been known for decades that BAME staff have experienced bullying and racism. (see chapter 2). Many experienced discriminations at the interviewing stage, during training and after qualifying as a doctor or nurse. Over and above the internal workings of medical and nursing schools there were other external factors at play. These were and are now in the era of the hostile environment, the overt hostility during the EU referendum and the state sponsored attack on British African-Caribbean's known as the Windrush scandal. Racism and bullying reared their heads again during the COVID- 19 crisis. National Centre Against Bullying (NACB) (no date) (21) defined bullying as an ongoing and deliberate misuse of power in relationships through repeated verbal, physical and/or social behaviour. It is intended to cause physical, social and/or psychological harm. This could involve an individual or a group abusing and/or misusing their power, or perceived power, over one and/or more persons. Victims feel unable to stop it from happening as they feel powerless. Bullying can happen in person, online, via various digital platforms and devices, and it can be obvious (overt) or hidden (covert). Bullying behaviour is repeated, or has the potential to be repeated, over time, for example, through sharing of digital records. Bullying of any form or for any reason can have immediate, medium and long-term effects on those involved, including bystanders. This can take many forms i.e. race, ethnicity, gender, disability, age, social class, sexuality, etc. Bullying can also happen from staff towards a more senior employee, a manager or an employer (this can be called 'upward bullying' or 'subordinate bullying'). It can be from one employee or group of employees. Examples of upward bullying can include showing continued disrespect, refusing to complete tasks, spreading rumours and/or doing things to make one seem unskilled or unable to do your job properly (Arbitration, Conciliation and Arbitration Service) (ACAS 2023) (22). Racism is defined as a belief that people differ along biological and genetic lines and that one's group is superior to another group. This belief is coupled with the power to negatively affect the lives of those perceived to be inferior. Its members believe that their race is mentally, physically, morally and culturally superior. Consequently, this group or groups believe they are entitled to special rights and privileges on a direct or institutional level. In the West there is a false belief that white people are "superior", relative to those who are not white. Racism can be manifested in many ways and for the purposes of this chapter only direct and institutional forms will be (briefly) discussed. Direct racism occurs when something obvious and blatant is said or done and people are treated less favourably due to their ethnicity or race. It is manifested on an interpersonal level and is embedded in the individuals' racist assumptions. This is promoted and sustained by the societal institutions like education, media, social policies, religion, popular media and other agencies. Institutional racism will be discussed in much more detail in the final chapter.

There was a strong sense that existing structural workplace inequality and the emotional burden of racial injustice were exacerbated during the pandemic. Jesuthasan et al revealed participants felt that increased COVID-19 vulnerability compounded their career advancement challenges. The pandemic provided an opportunity for 'unconscious bias' among management to manifest itself in career advancement opportunities given to non-ethnic minority staff. Of all the inequalities faced by BAME staff, COVID-19 became yet another hurdle they had to endure. One example illustrated that management under the cover of the chaos promoted white people. There was a strong view that the activities of Black Lives Matter raised uncomfortable questions among the workforce and as one person stated, "it felt that you were being attacked by all sides". Others pointed that there was lack of acknowledgement of one's vulnerability, in the sense that it was BAME people who were disproportionately impacted upon. There was an unasked question that if the virus was impacting on the white people, things would have been different. Participants reported feeling under pressure to continue front line working. This arose both from managers and an innate sense of duty with a sense of duty and

"Who was going to do the work".

Another related there was this whole thing about the

"Virus lasting 2 weeks max".

So many members of staff were harassed and told

"You have to go back, your 2 weeks are up".

If you are a nurse in a unit that is short-staffed and you turn up for work and they don't have the necessary PPE, you either get on with your job knowing that you're at high-risk or you become a problem (Jesuthasan et al). Ramamurthy et al added some BAME nurses felt harassed with phone calls every day while they were ill to find out when they were returning to work.

Elahi (2021) (23) concurred with Jesuthasan et al from a survey by the BMA. Dr Nagaul said there were "longstanding inequalities" in the NHS and career progression isn't great for BAME doctors. They tend to be in patient facing roles more than white doctors and more of them have been on the front line during the pandemic. Many of these doctors were afraid of speaking up due to fear of reprisals and implications for further employment. This was a huge factor especially for those on short term visa. People have spoken about pressure of work, but they don't want to say anything that might rock the boat. More than 700 doctors who participated in the research felt discriminated against by colleagues or managers during the pandemic. A further 700 said they felt bullied at work. Dr Ronx Ikharia supported the previous findings and added another specific element. There are about 20,000 Filipino nurses in the NHS, most have been actively recruited, paid their own fares and visa to get here. There is evidence that migrant workers were threatened with losing their jobs and visas if they do not accept redeployment to COVID-19 departments. Overseas workers were seen as commodities when they get us through recruitment from other countries to get to their land to "work as their slaves" (Ramamurthy et al). According to the Filipino Nurses Association many of these nurses work numerous shifts and were hardest hit by the pandemic. They were allocated along with other BAME staff to *"red"* wards where many patients were severely ill with the coronavirus. As one nurse stated,

"We don't find it easy in our hearts to say no" even if we have concerns about PPE. Another pointed out,

"I did not know what bullying was about until somebody said it".

Extracts from Ramamurthy et al added,

"You are here to work. I don't care if you die or not, I don't care if you are sick or not, just work".

"They don't care about us, no compassion, no understanding, no nothing. Just cold as ice or colder than ice".

The Filipino Association estimated that about 20 per cent of these nurses died during the pandemic and there is a strong suspicion that these deaths were related to work. ITN's largest survey of 4000 respondents at the time (15th May 2020) agreed and added of the 2000 respondents 84 per cent of BAME staff are more likely to be deployed on the front line and with lack of PPE, and do not speak out due to fear of being discriminated against. They do not feel represented at senior management level and their views are not heard. This is commonly referred to as the *"snowy white peaks"*. These are without doubt the manifestations of institutional racism. BAME staff suffered disproportionately compared to their white counterparts.

Ramamurthy et al study revealed the impact of racism. The findings of the study illustrated 59 per cent of BAME staff had experienced racism during their working lives that made it difficult for them to do their job. 53 per cent said racism impacted on their mental health. 36 per cent had left their job because of racism during their working lives. 33.4 per cent had been forced to take sick leave as a result of racism. All these are rooted in the very structure of the NHS and have been even since its inception.

There is a strong body of evidence to indicate that managers have and are responsible for discriminating against BAME staff. This has been going on for decades. Managers since the inception of the NHS, have been responsible for the recruitment and allocation of BAME staff to the "Cinderella" services, failure to provide adequate support, equal opportunities in promotion, and disproportionately referring them to the profession bodies. (See DHSS 1978, Hugman 1991, Torkington 1991, Ahmad 1993, Coker 2002, Batty 2020, Burnet et al 2020, and others in chapter 2). In my own experience as an ex-nurse, I witnessed how the grading system was unfairly managed. The system involved nurses being graded according to their skills and experiences. Grade "A" being the lowest and grade 'I' the highest at very senior managers. Many of my BAME colleagues were downgraded and their white counterparts with limited experience were allocated senior grades. Many BAME colleagues were stuck at 'F' grade with protected pay for two years. The white nurses progressed very quickly along the grades and became their managers. Consequently, many of my BAME colleagues retired at the earliest opportunity, others left to work in the private sector, and some were made redundant. Given this track record, it is of no surprise then that in many instances the managers failed in their duty of care towards their employees. It cannot be ruled out that the same managers who have been allocating BAME staff disproportionately to "red wards", providing some with ill-fitting or unsuitable PPE, coercing staff to "keep quiet and carry on" have been allocated the task of conducting risk assessment on the very same staff.

Conclusion

This chapter has discussed that numerous BAME staff in the NHS have succumbed from COVID- 19. During the first wave (March 2020 to July 2020) the alarm was raised when about 70 per cent of doctors who died were of BAME ethnicity. They were followed by a number of other staff mostly nurses. It is reported that around 20 per cent of Filipino nurses died during the time when COVID-19 was active. There is a recurring theme that account for the over-representation of BAME NHS staff deaths. There were accounts that many of these staff were not provided with suitable and appropriate PPE while they were actively engaged in their caring duties. There were repeated claims by the government that PPE was available for those who needed them most. Shortage was denied and it was seen as a distribution issue. This did not chime with emerging evidence from front line staff. Some purchased their own PPE from DIY stores and others were using plastic bin bags to protect themselves from being contaminated. Additionally, many PPE that arrived were out of date, wrongly labelled, and not fit for purpose. PPE was designed with no regard for the requirement of some BAME staff and was designed on the model of a white face and did not cater for those who wore a turban, head covering, or for those sporting a beard. Some reported that in some cases managers hid PPEs. Due to the high number of deaths, hospital trusts were required to conduct risk assessments on all staff and take appropriate actions to mitigate the risk factors for those who were deemed to be at increased risk. However, many claimed that the risk assessment was simply a paper exercise and were largely not acted upon. Risk assessment was not always followed by risk management. On occasions it was left for individuals to take the initiative and asked to be relocated to another area. These were other reasons as to why so many BAME staff died from COVID-19; they were delegated to high-risk areas and often with poor or unsuitable PPE. The other factor was that BAME staff are over-represented on front line and patient-facing roles. As a former front line nurse for seventeen years and lecturer for about twenty years, these are of no surprise to me. Since the inception of the NHS, BAME medical and nursing staff have always been sent to the unpopular areas by managers. I remember being sent to the wards with very high workloads. These would be areas with staff shortages and patients who needed intensive support. Had I been in clinical practice even as a lecturer, I would have been re-deployed by managers to areas with severely sick people with COVID-19. I have been reminded on many occasions that I was here "to work" and given disproportionate workloads compared to my white counterparts. What occurred during 2020 and beyond with the arrival of the virus, a well tried and tested method was implemented. White staff are mostly in management roles. This is still the case and is referred to as *"snowy white peaks"*. There is no doubt that many BAME staff were bullied and coerced to work, while white staff were given time off. Numerous BAME staff felt obliged to continue in their role due to sense of duty and were reluctant to speak out due to fear of reprisals and their impact on further employment. It is absolutely shocking that with so much evidence of bullying and racism in the NHS, which has been going on for decades, some managers who were themselves at the very heart of these activities and were allocating staff to high-risk areas were tasked to conduct risk assessments. There are shades of repeat of what was going on during both World Wars, when black and Asian soldiers were sent to the front line with limited training and equipment. They were used as cannon fodder. As discussed in previous chapter, Doyal and Pennell argued that BAME staff were both a disposable and reserve workforce. Hugman also pointed out that the echoes of colonialism are reproduced in health and care work and professionalism is going on in an atmosphere of racism. Torkington (1991) (24) argued that every organisation has its rules and regulations which informs and direct the way an organisation functions. The enforcement and interpretation of these rules and regulations are left in the hands of those who are in positions of power. All that is needed is to ensure that the rules and regulations are rigidly applied in the case of those against whom one wishes to discriminate. This form of racism is not only difficult to detect but also difficult to challenge.

The implication of various Race Relations Acts, equal opportunities policies and the duty of care to staff seemed to have been ignored or left out. Managers collectively failed to support their BAME staff when it was most needed. Senior managers have bestowed upon them much power and authority. This includes the power to act or not to act. Evidence suggests that as a collective group, managers decided to send BAME staff to the battlefield without suitable and appropriate PPE. When risk assessments were conducted the findings were not always followed by risk management. In 1995 Nolan identified Seven Principles of Public Life, which were and are selflessness, integrity, objectivity, accountability, openness, honesty and leadership. The Francis Report in 2013 after the Mid Staffordshire NHS Foundation Trust made 290 recommendations. Some are openness, transparency, cultural change in the NHS, compassionate caring and committed care, duty of candour and among others the freedom to speak out. All public officeholders are both servants of the public and stewards of public resources. All the evidence suggests that these principles have been collectively overlooked. There is little if any evidence of managers being challenged or held accountable for action and/or the commission of their actions. Consequently, there is no change in managers' behaviour and the same practice is repeated and again. The cycle remains operative and new staff will receive the same treatment. Is it any surprise that the NHS is and has been haemorrhaging staff? This of course is of no consequence. Shortfall is easily rectified. This has been the modus operandi of the NHS since the sixties. Recruit from overseas. It is quicker, cheaper and the entire process starts again. Status quo is maintained. These practices cannot be those of *'a few bad apples'*. The entire orchard has been planted in the soil that has been poisoned by the ideology of white superiority. This can only be seen as collective failure not unwitting activity. It is a well-crafted and well-executed system. The obvious question is if the NHS treats its most valuable resource in this way, what of patients, especially when COVID -19 was rampant?

CHAPTER 10
COVID-19 AND HEALTH INEQUALITIES

Serious and entrenched health inequalities existed well before the arrival of COVID-19. These were and are manifested in regional, gender, age and ethnicity. Much evidence indicated that social determinants are critical in the manifestations of these inequalities. These were exacerbated when the virus arrived in the backdrop of over a decade long austerity measures. In 1984, a WHO discussion document proposed a moving away from viewing health as a state and move towards a dynamic model that presented it as a process or a force. This was expanded in 1986 by the Ottawa Charter for Health Promotion. The University of Ottawa defined health as,

"The extent to which an individual or group is able to realize aspirations and satisfy needs, and to change or cope with the environment. Health is a resource for everyday life, not the objective of living; it is a positive concept, emphasizing social and personal resources, as well as physical capacities."

This definition implies some determinants are necessary for the maintenance of health. Ratcliff (2020) (1) argued that in the past two decades the WHO has emphasised the importance of social determinants of health. That is the way a particular society is constructed affects health. These are the drivers of the conditions of life, the political economy of health, power and politics. They influence the conditions of life and the impact on health outcomes. The determinants are suitable and affordable housing, low pollution levels, the income from and type of employment, access to occupational health, stress associated with the ability to pay bills, have access to suitable education, to green spaces and reduction of absolute and relative poverty[14]. Others are leisure facilities, affordable and suitable food, access to transport and health promotion. The other health determinants are social class, gender, age and ethnicity. The Black Report (1982) Health Divide (1987) Acheson Report (1995) and Marmot (2020) have discussed these extensively. They all concur that working class people, women, old people and those of BAME ethnicity have poorer health and life chances compared to affluent males and younger people. Ratcliff argued these are structural inequalities and are produced by society. She continued that the racial structure of society causes and reinforces sexism, classism, ageism and racism. BAME people face both direct and institutional racism constantly. There is a growing recognition that racism as a health determinant is understudied yet extremely important. All these determinants were compounded by austerity measures and continued to have a disproportionate impact on visible minorities. The first part of this chapter discusses the regional, age and gender inequalities and is followed with a detailed discussion on how BAME patients fared during the COVID-19 outbreak. It concludes by critiquing the responses by Public Health England and the Race Disparity Unit.

---

[14] **Absolute poverty** – is a condition where household income is below a necessary level to maintain basic living standards (food, shelter, housing).

Relative poverty – A condition where household income is a certain percentage below median income. For example, the threshold for relative poverty could be set at 50% of median incomes (or 60%) Economics Help (2019) Definition of absolute and relative poverty.
https://www.economicshelp.org/blog/glossary/definition-of-absolute-and-relative-poverty/ Accessed 15/6/2023.

As regards to health inequalities the concept of inverse care law is as true today as it was in 1971. These long-standing inequalities have been exacerbated by the continuing years of austerity. An indelible mark has been left in the health of those living in most deprived areas. There is no blow-by-blow discussion on statistics but rather to gather a collective view that has emerged during the crisis in England. As the virus raged, it became clear that it was affecting people in different ways.

There were regional variations throughout the country with disproportionately affected the North of England (Northwest, Northeast, Yorkshire, and Humber regions). This increased regional ill-health and economic inequalities. Northerners were more likely to die from COVID-19 and spent nearly six more weeks in lockdowns. They suffered worse mental health and were made poorer than the rest of England during the first year of the pandemic (NHSA) (2021) (2). People living the North had a 17 per cent higher mortality rate from COVID-19 than those in the rest of England. Their mortality rate due to all causes was 14 per cent higher. About half of the increased COVID-19 mortality in the North and two-thirds of the increased all-cause mortality were explained by potentially preventable higher deprivation and worse pre-pandemic health. Mortality rates in care homes in the North of England were 26 per cent higher than the rest of England and 10 per cent more hospital beds were occupied by patients than in the rest of England. In terms of restrictions on average, people living in the North had 41 more days of the harshest restrictions than people in the rest of the country. They also experienced a larger drop in mental well-being, more loneliness, and were prescribed higher rates of antidepressants. Public Health England (PHE) reported that London, as well as the East and West Midlands, were significantly affected.

Conversely, the Southwest [15] experienced the lowest levels of morbidity and mortality.

The Office of National Statistics (ONS) (2021) (3) noted between March 2020 and January 2021 in England and Wales there was an almost 18 per-cent difference in the total number of COVID-19 related deaths for men (63,700) and women (53,300). In the early stages of the pandemic, particularly between 1st March and 30th of April 2020, the difference was even starker: 30 per cent more men (21,600) than women (16,600) died in the UK. There were over 38,200 deaths involving COVID-19 during that period, and men accounted for around 57 per cent. As the year progressed, the difference in the number of deaths between men and women narrowed until the end of September 2020, when the gap between them began to open again. This peaked in the week ending 22nd January 2021.

McIntyre et al (2022) (4) suggested the elderly (75 years and over) were also adversely impacted by the pandemic. It has taken the greatest toll on them: across the UK since the start of the pandemic more than seven in ten registered deaths have been among those aged 75 or older. Meanwhile, deaths among those aged forty-four or younger made up of less than 2 per-cent of the total. The proportion of deaths made up by older people seems to have changed over the course of the pandemic. It is worthy to note that the above inequalities are discussed without making any reference to culture or genetics.

In March 2020 the National Health Service England (NHSE) (5) ordered that hospitals should urgently discharge all in-patients who were deemed medically fit. This meant elderly people, with a view to maximising the use of the Care Homes which were predominantly in

---

[15] Southwest includes Cornwall, Dorset, Devon, Bristol, Gloucestershire, Somerset and Wiltshire.

the private sector. It is well-established that many elderly people died in these care homes.

Spencer and Yorke (2022) (6) stated,

"By April 2020 the risk of death for a resident in care home was 17 times higher than someone of the same age living at home. By the end of May 2020 many deaths have been recorded in social care".

Huffpost (2022) (7) referred to a court case brought by two women whose fathers died from the virus. They challenged the health secretary and PHE over the policy. The barrister told the court that between March 2020 and June 2020 more than 20,000 elderly or disabled residents in care homes died from COVID-19 in England and Wales. That death toll should not and need not have happened, the barrister argued. The spokesperson for one of the bereaved families said,

"I lost my father in a care home back in April 2020. We kept him there because we had been told that no one in the care home had COVID-19, and he would be safe, but we learnt later from the staff that 27 patients had died from the virus there". "We've always known that our loved ones were thrown to the wolves by the government and claims made by the health secretary that 'a protective ring' round care homes was "a sickening lie".

The High Court ruled that the government's action for sending hospital patients into care homes at the start of the pandemic was unlawful. This means that it is not authorised by law as no such law has been passed. Many of these elderly people were sent to care homes without a negative COVID-19 test. Duncan (2021) (8) argued more people died of COVID-19 in care homes in England and Wales in the second wave of the pandemic rather than in the first. Data from the ONS indicated while the rise in coronavirus deaths among care home residents were much higher during the first wave (between March and September 2020), the number and proportion of COVID-19 deaths were higher in the second wave from September to April 2021. This may be due to more testing during the second wave. The exact number of deaths during the first wave is disputable as many who were sent to care homes were not tested for COVID-19. In essence it is not possible to argue with any accuracy where and how these elderly people contracted the virus and subsequently died from it. While the exact numbers may be debated, there is no denying the fact that many elderly people were sent to care homes, and they died there often on their own. It is not clear if data on gender and ethnicity were extrapolated from these deaths.

COVID-19 and its impact on BAME people

During the first wave (24 March 2020-4 July 2020) the warning signs were that all was not well with morbidity and mortality rates of BAME people. It became a recurring theme throughout the daily ministerial briefings. There was an over-representation of BAME people in morbidity and mortality, and diverse ethnic groups were impacted differently. The Chief Medical Officer for England seemingly surprised by these findings during the very early stages of the pandemic commissioned the PHE to "understand the extent that *ethnicity* impacted upon risk and outcome". I am not a statistician so my discussion will be from a sociological and lay perspective. The PHE produced its initial findings in Beyond the Data in June 2020 (PHE) [1] (9). It focussed primarily on *ethnicity* as a determinant of health. This was a reductionist way of analysing a very complex phenomenon. By focussing on *ethnicity,* it ignored the deleterious impact over the years of austerity, the wider socio-economic and other determinants of health like racism that have had and are still having a disproportionate impact on BAME people. PHE produced another report in August 2020 [2] (10) to highlight the over-representation of BAME people in morbidity and mortality from the virus. Both reports concur that the highest age standardised diagnosis rates were in people of Black ethnic groups and the lowest in people of white ethnic groups. The survival rate of people of Bangladeshi ethnicity was around twice the risk of death when compared to people of white ethnicity. The other minority ethnic groups had between 10-50 per cent higher risks of death when compared to the white British. They suggested,

"This is opposite of what is seen in previous years, when the all-cause mortality rates are lower in Asian and Black ethnic groups".

This statement is not supported by any references, elaborated or explained. This can be challenged on at least two perspectives. The critical determinants of health have consistently been associated with poor health. These became exponentially worse during over fourteen years of austerity measures, and they all concur that BAME people are and have been disproportionately impacted compared to their white counterparts. Given that most BAME people live in poverty, deprived areas, in poor housing, poorly paid employment, live in highly polluted areas, experience various forms and levels of racism; and have questionable trust in particularly primary care, it follows that BAME would have the worst health outcomes. These would be reflected in high morbidity and mortality. The other perspective is that there is considerable evidence that BAME are underserved by most if not all aspects of health provision. Some of these have been discussed above in mental health, elderly care and maternity care provision. Furthermore, the Black Report (1982), Acheson (2005), CMO report

(1992), Marmot (2016), and Ratcliff (2020) provided robust evidence for decades that BAME people have experienced and still experiencing worse morbidity and mortality in most if not all aspects of health.

The June 2020 PHE report points out that genetics were not included in the review. After reviewing a number of books and general health documents the question of genetics does not seem to appear when the health concerns of the white population is discussed. Ahmad (1993) (11) argued for black people the focus is exclusively on cultures, genetics and metabolism meant being different and therefore inferior. In June 2020 the PHE held a stakeholder engagement. Many were personally affected by the high death rates and stated that COVID-19 has exacerbated long-standing and entrenched health inequalities. These were due to upstream factors and are due to structural and societal inequalities. These are socio-economic political factors which in turn have impact on all if not most determinants of health. These have been exacerbated by over fourteen years of austerity which have disproportionately affected the life chances of most BAME people. The lack of trust and being underserved by health and social services has been consistently highlighted. There was call for continuous community engagement to build trust and carry out research with the active participation of the community. Health promotion information needed to be developed and should take into consideration the linguistic and cultural make up of the given community. Stakeholders made specific reference to the importance of addressing racism and discrimination. Of note, the PHE report in August of 2020 does not make any reference to the stakeholders' views. Nor did it discuss racism and discrimination but referred, albeit briefly, to a variety of socio-economic and political determinants of health. It made a very sweeping statement by way of "explaining" why BAME people were disproportionately impacted by the virus. It stated, "People for BAME groups are also more likely than white people to be born abroad, which means they may face additional barriers in accessing services that are created by for example cultural and language differences". As a BAME person who has lived here for over fifty years, I am not sure what aspect of my culture or language has placed additional barriers in accessing health care. All the obstacles I faced have been placed by people and policies of institutions. More importantly it is well-documented that BAME people have lived here for centuries and especially since 1948, the same year the NHS was created. There is very little evidence that the NHS (and other institutions) have made concerted effort to address the health needs of BAME people, despite many were recruited to prop up the NHS itself. An explanation of this could well be that there is and has been a poor representation of BAME people in very senior management roles. It is true that some BAME people have recently migrated to Britain and this ought to be factored in the development of appropriate and sensitive care provision. The statement falls in the usual trap of blaming BAME people for being infected and lays the blame in our place of birth, culture and language. The failure of the NHS and other institutions to address our needs is ignored yet again. We are seen as being the problem and/or having the problem.

During the start of the vaccination period between 8 December 2020 and December 2021 the approximate end of the second wave, people from all ethnic minority groups except the Chinese group and women in the white other ethnic groups, had a higher rate of death involving COVID-19 compared with the white British population (ONS 2022) (12). During the same period, the rate of death involving COVID-19 was the highest for the Bangladeshi ethnic group (5.0 times greater that the white British group for males, and 4.5 greater for females), followed by the Pakistani (3.1 for males, 2.6 for females) and Black African (2.4 for males, 1.7 for females) ethnic groups. Since the start of the third wave of the coronavirus pandemic (from 13 June 2021 onwards) the rate of death involving COVID-19 was higher for most ethnic minority groups. The exception was Chinese people, men from the mixed ethnic group and women from the white other ethnic groups. The risk remains highest for the Bangladeshi ethnic group which was 4.4 and 5.2 times greater than all the white British ethnic group for males and females respectively. Nafilyan et al (2021) (13) supported most of the findings.

Scobie, Spencer, and Raleigh (2021) (14) highlighted another long-standing problem. After examining Hospital Episode Statistics from 2010-2011 to 2019-2020, they found that many health-related datasets do not routinely record patient ethnicity. Consequently, ethnicity within hospital records was used. Unfortunately, miscoding in hospital data meant that estimates of COVID-19 infection, hospitalisation, and death could be over-or under-counted in minority ethnic and white groups. Further analysis found data gathering problems included incomplete codes, inconsistent use of codes, an increase of patients recorded as "not known" "not stated" or "other". This impeded reliable analysis of ethnic differences and data quality problems affecting minority ethnic patients. The lack of comprehensive, high-quality data on health and mortality by ethnicity is a significant obstacle to understanding ethnic inequalities in health. This makes it difficult to assess and plan how the diverse health needs of different ethnic groups can be addressed. Furthermore, death certificates do not record ethnicity; it records place of birth. However, there is no doubting which ethnic groups were affected by the virus. In the words of a clinician

"You can't argue with the number of BAME people who are on COVID-19 wards, Intensive care units and dying".

The Beyond the Data PHE report June 2020 prompted some strong reactions from various organisations. King's Fund (2020) (15) reinforced the fact that these forms of inequalities have been known for many years but there has been disappointingly little effort over the last decade to address them and improve people's health. It had taken a global pandemic to shine a light on these deeply and entrenched inequalities. Moore (2020) (16) in an exclusive report argued that the government censored BAME COVID-19 risk review and suggested that key sections were removed from the PHE's review of June 2020. Health Service Journal (HSJ) referred to the section of the implication of structural racism and discrimination. These views were collated from over one thousand organisations and individuals. According to the source that provided information to HSJ, the report was delayed in order not to stoke racial tension. The Department of Health and Social Care denied this allegation. The statement can be challenged on two fronts. Firstly, BAME have and are still suffering from major health inequalities. These and among others are in mental health, maternity and childcare, elderly care and haemoglobinopathies (See chapter 3). There is no evidence to suggest any of these entrenched and deep-seated inequalities led to any *racial tension*. Secondly, it implied that BAME people and communities would react spontaneously and cause *racial tension*. Has the latter become a victim to the age-old stereotype that BAME people are impulsively aggressive and not able to articulate their views in an appropriate manner? In the final analysis structural racism which is a significant determinant of health does not feature in the August PHE review of 2020. There was no disputing the fact that BAME people were significantly impacted by COVID-19 in both morbidity and mortality. The causes were identified by many long-standing socio-economic factors but there was no discussion as to how and what led to these. There is a distinct impression that PHE has not placed these in a much wider socio-political, historical, and economic context.

The Office for National Statistics (ONS) published two further reports on 26 July 2021 (ONS) (17) and 19 August 2021 (ONS) (18). They discussed ethnic differences in the life expectancy and mortality from **selected** causes in England and Wales from 2011-2014. Data on morbidity in mental health, maternity and peri-natal mortality were not included. It based its findings on **experimental analysis** of ethnic differences in life expectancy and cause-specific mortality of cancer and circulatory conditions in England and Wales based on 2011 Census and death registrations. The **estimated national** findings were during the pre-pandemic period of 2011-2014. The August report was still based on experimental data with Dementia and Alzheimer's added to the list. The conclusion was both males and females in the white and mixed ethnic groups had lower life expectancy at birth than all other ethnic groups; the Black African group had statistically significant higher life expectancy than most groups. My first reaction was a statement I have heard many times in relation to interpreting statistics. It can be designed to support any "fact" to prove a particular assertion. It is still questionable as to who made this comment, but Mark Twain appear to be credited with these words,

"There are 3 kinds of lies: lies, damned lies and statistics".

Sandercock et al (SMC 2021) (19) drilled down on the data and posits that the sample was made of 96 per cent of white people which would be an accurate representation of the white population. On the other hand, joining the numbers of black African women and Asian 'Other' men constituted only .5 per cent of the population studied. Therefore, the extent to which this represents the entire group needs to be challenged. Nazroo (2021) (20) argued these experimental statistics should be treated with caution and not considered to be robust or conclusive, and no assertion on ethnic inequalities should be based solely on them. Mortality rates, Nazroo suggested, requires a count of the number of people who died (within a particular time frame) and the size of the population they came from. To put it simply, the number of deaths divided by population size. The problem is we don't know the size of each ethnic group and furthermore the 2011 census is ten years out of date. Many ethnic minorities or BAME people could have migrated out of England and Wales since then. Nazroo commented,

"There are important concerns that should be taken into account when interpreting the experimental statistics on ethnic differences in life expectancy and mortality rates produced by the ONS. It is likely that the key problems discussed will have led to an underestimate of mortality rates and an overestimate of life expectancy for ethnic minority people compared with white people".

ONS records of July and August 2021 indicated that 90 per cent of black Africans and 95 per cent of other Asian deaths were recorded as "immigrants" to Britain. There is a general view that immigrants are healthier than the local people as all are subject to strict medical examination before they can apply for a visa to enter other countries. I had to undergo chest x-ray, blood tests, dental examination, and immunisation against infections before applying for a visa. This is called the "healthy immigrant effect". This group are unlikely to use the health services at least in the initial stages. There is also a view that their health would diminish over time. The reason is these "immigrants" may adopt unhealthy lifestyles of the "natives". However, another perspective is that the decline in the health of the 'healthy immigrant' could be due to the wider social and structural racism which will impact on almost all determinants of health. It is well documented that direct and institutional racism impacts on every aspect of life. Furthermore, these 'healthy immigrants' once in the country would have limited information to access health care, advice and guidance about health issues, education, social care, and a host of health and well-being agencies. The role of health institutions is to mitigate for these issues. They may be healthy on arrival, but it is questionable as to how long this would last. The idea of the healthy immigrant effect is in itself very contentious and needs to be treated with much caution. Another difficulty was that those who are deemed healthy on arrival may be people of white ethnicity, so their life chances may well be very different to those who are not white. Both Sandercock et al and Nazroo suggested again that death certificates did not record ethnicity during COVID-19 era. Linking data to the 2011 census cannot be perfect. This is the first time this statistical analysis has been used, and the result must be seen as experimental, and may well need changes. Statistical data tells us what may be occurring but not why differences occur. The ONS publications of July and August 2021 do concede that the experimental statistics are in a testing phase and findings need further research. As a layperson I am not sure as to why cancer, cardiovascular illnesses, dementia and Alzheimer's which are not infective disorders, are being compared to COVID-19. There is also an assumption that the "white" group is a homogenous group.

There are other contributory factors which predisposed BAME people to COVID-19. Over and above the long-standing and entrenched inequalities faced by BAME people, other determinants have contributed to the disproportionate impact on this section of the community. As discussed above, various studies have indicated that BAME people suffer disproportionately from various disorders. It is beyond doubt that black men are more likely to be (mis)diagnosed with having serious mental illness, detained and given physical forms of treatment, women of Asian, Black or mixed-race ethnicity have an elevated risk of maternal death is more than four times higher than for white women. Mortality rates from coronary heart disease are higher than average for people born in South Asia and lower for those born in the Caribbean. South Asians tend to experience central obesity and insulin resistance which may pre-dispose them to diabetes and coronary heart disease. Overall, people from minority ethnic groups are more likely to describe their health as "fair" or "poor" than the ethnic majority. It is generally agreed that co-morbidities may well have played a role in the high number of BAME people being adversely impacted.

There are other factors to be considered. ONS (2020) (21) highlighted a number of occupational hazards that led to an increased exposure to the virus. Black and Asian men are more likely to work in occupations that have a high frequency of contact with members of the public. They are in transport as taxi, and bus drivers, chefs (who are mostly Bangladeshi and Pakistani men), security officers, cleaners, shopkeepers, delivering post, mail sorters, domestics, work in clothing factories, and key workers. Many are more likely to use public transport. These occupations are poorly paid, and no work means no pay. This results in more poverty. Most if not all, they cannot work from home. The Race Disparity Unit (2020), (22) (2021) (23), (2021) (24), (2021) (25) published four quarterly reports between October 2020 and December 2021. They set out the action plan taken to

"Consider why the virus has had such a disproportionate impact on people from ethnic minority groups".

It worked across other government documents to achieve its objectives.

The recommendations can be summarised as follows:

- There should be more research to build an evidence base to get a better understanding of what is driving those disparities. No doubt universities and academics would be very keen to conduct even more research on ethnic minorities.

- It placed much emphasis on 'Community Engagement' with the purpose of promoting the uptake of vaccines. This was to be achieved by building trust between the local communities and health institutions. The aim was to 'Promote Healthy Living', to translate health promotion information in community languages and use different media to ensure that these messages reach all sections of the community.

- Make use of the local voluntary and grass roots organisations as advocates to promote the uptake of COVID-19 vaccines and challenge 'misinformation' in the community. Ironically these very organisations have been almost decimated by the decade long austerity measures, and consequently many had their funding cut or reduced.

- They proposed to 'find out' why Pakistani and Bangladeshi people were even more severely impacted upon by the virus.

- The other recommendations were more about NHS and health organisations. They were to monitor the impact of their policies, mandatory recording of patient's ethnicity in medical records and death certificates and harmonise ethnicity classification.

- The final points in the last report were "we now know" and makes reference to "avoid stigmatising" ethnic minority groups, encouraging these groups to engage in clinical trials, and University of Oxford have identified the gene responsible for doubling the risk of respiratory failure from COVID-19 which apparently is carried by 61 per-cent of people from South Asian ancestry.

The other suggestions were about community engagement with the purpose to 'educate' 'promote healthy living' and most of all to increase the uptake of the vaccine. I, as a person of "South Asian ancestry", need to have an advocate, be represented by community leaders and grass roots workers. I must be re-educated about the benefits of the vaccine and the transmission of the virus. I belong to a "hard to reach group", live in communities, and above all, am not an individual. I have done all these on my own volition. These are ideas others have of my "inferiority". Many stereotypes about South Asian people have already been discussed. We were and are seen as being less than human, that cannot be trusted and viewed with much suspicion. We as South Asians have already been "othered". The quarterly reports made frequent reference to avoid stigmatising ethnic minorities but the entire concept of 'community engagement and educating people' ended up doing exactly that. These modes of thinking are not new. Black, Asian, and other minority soldiers were subject to these ideologies during both World Wars and even before that. The ideologies seem to re-appear during times of crisis, be it political or otherwise. The PHE reports and quarterly reports gave a distinct impression that we as BAME people have recently landed in Britain. The powers that be suddenly noticed during COVID-19 that many Bangladeshi and Pakistani people are in front line work like taxi drivers, bus drivers, shopkeepers, key workers, and other jobs. Black African and Caribbean people, especially men work in the security industry. It took a pandemic to direct the attention of policymakers to this. The question is how long will this last? The irony is that all this information has been available for decades, but individuals and institutions simply ignored them.

Many reports have suggested that continuous and meaningful engagement should have been made between health providers and the local community decades ago. If this was held regularly on the terms of the local people, it would have generated trust and facilitate access to health and a whole host of useful and sensitive health provision. As in the June PHE report, stakeholders were willing to undertake research in partnership and collaboration with health providers. On an operational level, most community and grass roots organisations which were critical in gaining first-hand information from these communities were decimated during the fourteen years of austerity. Many had their funding cut or significantly reduced. Currently building trust will be a serious challenge on several grounds. There are extensive discussions as to the services are provided to BAME people in mental health, maternity care, elderly care, and among others haemoglobinopathies. BAME people also experience much difficulty in accessing GPs and their level of satisfaction with this service is rated well below the satisfaction compared to their white counterparts.

It's in my genes or jeans!

The final quarterly report of December 2021 boldly states under the category of *we now know* argued that over and above occupation, living in multigenerational households and living in areas of high deprivation, another factor is at play. Research by

"University of Oxford has identified the gene responsible for doubling the risk of respiratory failure from COVID-19 which is apparently carried by 61% of people from South Asian ancestry".

The gene is also carried by 15 per cent of those with white European backgrounds. It changes the way the lungs respond to infection. Not being a geneticist, I am not able to comment on this discovery. As a layperson, I can ask a few questions. The term South Asian is a diverse and includes people from India, Pakistan, Bangladesh, Nepal, Bhutan, Maldives, and among others Sri Lanka. South Asians have migrated around the world for centuries, especially during various periods of colonisation when many were transported to countries around the world. It would be interesting to see what would happen when people of South Asian (who have this gene) marry people who do not have the *gene*. Many South Asians married non-South Asians so we assume that this *gene* may well be present in other ethnic groups. Equally, if *this gene* was already there it would follow that South Asians would have been the most over-represented people in morbidity and mortality. All the data during the first wave of the virus was according to the 'Disparities in the risk and outcome from COVID-19' of August indicated that death rates were higher for Black and Asian groups compared to white ethnic groups. This changed during the second wave and the disproportionate impact on Pakistani and Bangladeshi people became apparent. On the face of it the *gene* was absent during the first wave and appeared during the second wave? It is also noteworthy that the Oxford research concluded that the increased risk could be cancelled by the vaccine. However, the Oxford scientist use the term "could" often indicating that this is not definite. Rutherford (2020) (26) argued that although academic papers are published in reputable papers via the process of peer review, is the standard way of disseminating research; this is not a marker of some gold standard of truth. It is a signifier that the research is of a standard worthy of further academic discussion. Scientists disagree all the time about results, or the techniques used. It is perfectly possible for papers in a reputable journal to be flawed. According to Devlin (2021) (27) other scientists cautioned that the findings needed further confirmation, and genetic explanations should not overshadow other more potentially, more significant, socio-economic risk factors faced by ethnic minorities. These include increased risk of exposure and unequal access to healthcare. Devlin referred to Dr Nazrul Islam of Oxford University's Nuffield Department of Population of Health highlighted that some ethnicities are not well represented in the large genetic database used to determine the prevalence of this gene. He argued it provides an easy gateway for policymakers to say, "it's genetics, we can't do anything".

On a personal level, I am of South Asian ancestry and have been fortunate to have a good job with a reasonable pension and live in a reasonable area. If I was a key worker, living in a poorer area, with high levels of deprivation, poor and overcrowded housing, polluted air, poor pay, and have a health issue, this would happen to me: I would be community engaged, need an advocate, educated in healthy living, disease transmission and given the vaccine. I would then be sent to the environment that affected my health even before COVID-19 arrived. I will become invisible again. My health needs, which were impacted by the social determinants, would be ignored till the next health emergency and/or another pandemic.

The suggestion of more research needs to be challenged. There is an assumption that research is value and culture free. Ahmad explained research is usually a medium through which solutions are found for a particular problem. He suggested that research problems do not exist in a vacuum. They are shaped within particular social, economic, professional, theoretical, ideological and historical contexts. BAME people have always been viewed as "problems" for centuries especially in health-care terms. This has prompted several research initiatives and has become a major health industry. However, its benefits to ethnic minorities in terms of understanding illness or improving healthcare are minimal. Ahmad continued most research have adopted an uncritical acceptance of the medical model and tended to operate within frameworks provided by the powerful definitions of doctors. Research was divorced from action and this led to more research by predominantly white and some BAME researchers which made little difference to BAME peoples' lives. There was an overemphasis on culture at the expense of power relations and structures including racism. 'Cultures' were and are still seen as static, inferior, deviant, or pathological, so that health issues tended to be explained in terms of "blame the victim". Scott (1999) (28) provided some insights as to how research should interpret data about ethnicity. They argued that the use of ethnicity data superficially may contribute to perpetuating ethnic inequalities rather than simply describing them. Focussing exclusively on ethnicity can obscure the complex pathways linking macroeconomics, social and public policies that impact on the daily lives of BAME people. Differences in the risk and outcome faced by different ethnic people can only be understood and addressed if analysis is interpreted in the context of how lives are lived and experienced. This includes experience of structural, institutional, and interpersonal (direct) discrimination rooted in racism. Proposed explanations for ethnic differences in risk and outcomes for COVID-19 should be tested with data, and with reference to the testimony of the minority ethnic groups concerned. Studying ethnicity is a complex area and working in partnership with representatives from the affected minority people will help to improve understanding and make research more useful to both these communities and those seeking to reduce inequality.

Ahmad (1993) also noted that health research must be set within a broad context. Ideas of white superiority were developed and well supported by pseudoscience, media, religion, and among others politicians. These ideas were very apparent in the way black and Asian soldiers were seen as inferior and not to be trusted or relied upon during both World Wars and throughout the colonial and post-colonial era. Health, illness and healthcare have been and are structured within social relationships, shaped by historical developments and contemporary social economic realities, and mediated through professional ideology. Racism in medical research cannot be analysed in isolation from a wider discussion on racial oppression and its historical context. PHE, ONS and Quarterly reports discussed very briefly the wider social determinants which may well have significant impact on the contraction of COVID-19 and how BAME people were disproportionately affected by it. They made some references to health determinants like occupation, geography, demography, socio-economic characteristics, deprivation, poverty, household composition, comorbidities and other contributing factors. However, there is no discussion on how these social determinants occur and the brief reference to racism did not appear after the June 2020 PHE report. This represents a blunt denial of all the century's long factors that have been instrumental in creating these social determinants of health and have disproportionately impacted upon BAME people. Another major limitation was the PHE and ONS reports failed to contextualise these inequalities in the wider historical perspective like colonialism and the ideology of white superiority. These have inevitably seeped into every aspect of social policy and include the NHS.

It was clear from the very outset that health institutions were determined to lay the blame at the door of the very people who were disproportionately impacted by the virus. The concept of victim-blaming has a long history in Britain. During 1902-1913 an outbreak of infectious disease which affected Afro-Asians broke out in Kenya during the British colonial days. Instead of acting to redress the appalling overcrowding which perpetuated the infection, the medical department simply imposed a blockade so that the infection would not reach the affluent areas occupied by white population. The appalling overcrowding was due to the British policy; cram as many people in and provide housing which was unfit for habitation Doyal (1979) (29). This ideology still underpins the provision of health services to this day.

Conclusion

This chapter has discussed the extent to which serious and entrenched inequalities in health was well identified before the arrival of COVID-19. There were regional inequalities wherein the northern regions experiencing more morbidity and mortality. Older men were disproportionately impacted upon compared to women, and socio-economic factors were central in the manifestations of these inequalities. Many elderly people were discharged from NHS facilities to care homes with no test to indicate if they were infected with the virus. Many died, often with no loved one with them. This was a blatant form of institutional ageism. Soon after the virus arrived it became obvious that BAME people were seriously impacted both in morbidity and mortality. During the early phase morbidity rates were higher for Black ethnic groups and the lowest in white ethnic groups. Death rates were higher for Black and Asian ethnic groups when compared to white ethnic groups. This changed in August 2020 when the PHE reported that people of Bangladeshi and Pakistani ethnicity had twice the number of deaths when compared to people of white ethnicity. Both PHE reports of June and August made a very controversial remark. Both suggested that this is the opposite of what is seen in previous years when the all-cause mortality rates were lower in Asian and Black ethnic groups. The Chief Medical Officer seemingly taken aback by these revelations decided to "understand" the extent that ethnicity impacts upon risk and outcomes. A stakeholder event was held and the June PHE reported on its findings. The key themes where entrenched inequalities were decades in the making and structural racism was the root cause of socio-economic, political and health inequalities. The August report made no reference to the stakeholder's meeting or the thorny subject of racism. The PHE was absolutely determined not to include the existence of racism as a significant determinant of health. They focussed exclusively on ethnicity and made superficial reference to the socio-political and historical factors of deprivation, environment, and the employment of BAME people. More worryingly, the ONS discussed ethnic differences in the life expectancy and mortality from *selected* causes in England and Wales from 2011-2014. It based its findings on *experimental analysis* of ethnic differences in life expectancy and cause-specific mortality of cancer and circulatory conditions in England and Wales based on 2011 Census and death registrations. The *estimated national* findings were during the pre-pandemic period of 2011-2014. These were strongly challenged by some academics on several grounds. Data on ethnicity was poorly recorded as death certificates did not collect the patients' ethnicity. Some data was compared with the 2011 census would be a decade out of date. The information was based on selected cases are experimental and estimated and should be treated with caution.

The quarterly reports focussed on educating the local community by using community engagement, local grass roots, and faith leaders. The purpose was to promote the uptake of the COVID-19 vaccine and avoid transmission, especially in multigenerational households. £30 million were allocated to these activities. If this sum was spent well before the pandemic arrived by actively engaging with the local community in an ongoing basis and making us feel part of the solution, it can only be assumed that much pain, suffering, morbidity and mortality could have been avoided. The entire plan was reactive, and after many people has suffered. The stable door was shut after the horse had already bolted. In the last quarterly report, it argued that a gene had been identified that is present in 61 per cent of people of South Asian ancestry. This discovery should also be treated with great caution as it does not indicate any form of certainty.

There is no doubt that the government machinery had one main objective. It failed to consider the root causes: the socio-historical and economic factors that have impacted on BAME people for centuries. The existence and manifestation of institutional and direct racism was absent from the entire debate. All the historical and contemporary evidence has been completely ignored. It was and is easier to blame BAME people for contracting the infection rather than examining the social and health determinants that made them sick in the first place. There was constant reference to the systematic lack of the collection of ethnicity data. In 2005 the DOH produced a Practical Guide for ethnic monitoring in the NHS, but there has been and is still concerted resistance to collect and analyse inpatient ethnicity data. No data collection meant no information, which in turn becomes an excuse for no action. Instead, smokescreens like selected, experimental and estimated data and the discovery of a gene are all used to obscure the real causes of high morbidity and mortality of BAME people from COVID-19. The government has and is engaging in active denial. There is another example when the government actively engaged in such activity. A case in point is the Commission for Race and Ethnic Disparities (CRED) April 2021.

CHAPTER 11
CRED REPORT FACT OR FICTION?

This chapter discusses and provides a critique of the findings of the government's sponsored report in the realm of race and ethnic disparities. The background is as follows: In 2016, 17.4 million people voted for Brexit, and 14 million voted for Boris Johnson, providing him with an eighty-two-seat majority. He became the prime minister after that. In 2020 while COVID-19 was rampant, another event occurred in USA. This was the killing of George Floyd[16] and it sparked uprisings across Britain and around the world. People of all ages and ethnicities were protesting about the killing. They argued that this event underscored the existence of direct and institutional racism in the police in the USA and this had implications in Britain. The government was taken aback by this popular movement as it was supported by many sections of the community. Black, Asian, white, and other minorities marched holding posters labelled "Black Lives Matter". The anger of the crowds was palpable and was well captured by various media channels. I have a different take on the reaction to the killing of Floyd. The way in which he was killed was horrendous to say the least. A police officer had his knee on the neck of Floyd for about nine minutes and forty seconds. A disproportionate amount of

---

[16] On the evening of 25 May 2020, white Minneapolis police officer Derek Chauvin kills George Floyd, a Black man, by kneeling on his neck for almost 10 minutes. The death, recorded by bystanders, touched off what is possibly the largest protest movement in the U.S. history and a nationwide reckoning on race and policing.

force was placed on his neck, and it caused him to stop breathing. This entire episode was captured on camera. The graphic images caused an international outcry. This would be a totally normal reaction. However, when many people die every day from poverty, deprivation, lack of suitable housing, and other forms of state brutality there is little by way of revulsion. Most do not get any media coverage.

The government response was very different to the protesters. It began a concerted and determined campaign to underplay the existence of racism in Britain. The then Prime Minister decided to "change the narrative" and he launched a plan to achieve just that. A Commission was created in July 2020. Its objective was to investigate race and ethnic *disparities* in the UK and why, to thoroughly examine the reason so many disparities persist and what needed to be done to eliminate or mitigate them. The project was launched when COVID-19 was rampant. The Commission on Race and Ethnic Disparities (CRED) (RDU 2021) (1) was chaired by Dr Tony Sewell and its report was published in March 2021. The composition of CRED was made up of ten commissioners drawn from a variety of fields spanning space scientist, business, education, economics, broadcasting, medicine, legal voluntary sector, and policing. None of these commissioners appeared to have in-depth knowledge of race relations, critical social policy or the racial politics of health. Nine were from ethnic minority backgrounds, a point frequently used by some to imply that they are representative of BAME people and more absurdly that they provide 'credibility' to the conclusion of the report. This is a stereotypical form of thinking. It implied that a few members of Black, Asian and minority ethnic people would represent the views of the majority.

This appointment did not chime well with some campaigners. Turnnidge (2020) (2) argued that Dr Sewell, a former teacher and international education consultant, had in 2013 worked with the then

Prime Minister Boris Johnson when he was the Mayor of London. In 2010, Sewell said: *"Much of the supposed evidence of institutional racism is flimsy."* He also suggested that the root cause of knife crime and gang culture among Black youths was absent fathers, citing figures showing that about 50 per cent of Black children grow up without a father. To others it confirmed a widely held view that the establishment is simply paying lip service to [the] deeply entrenched systemic problem of racism that exists in state institutions and society.

The key report's findings were that racism exists and criticised anti-racist activity. UK it argued, is not rigged against minorities, racism is not the main cause of inequalities or disparities, and social media "amplifies racist views". The report is critical of the term BAME and there should be praise for *immigrant optimism*. Education is seen as the *success story* for UK minorities, and there should be shame and pride in British history and family is the foundation stone of success. The report stated that institutional racism "does not exist" and is being liberally used, often to describe any circumstances in which difference in outcome between racial and ethnic groups exists in an institution without evidence to support such claims. It pointed out that in many cases ethnic minorities are doing better that the majority white people. CRED agreed that racism exists in Britain, but institutional racism does not. This was not a total surprise to many as the chairperson and the head of policy unit at Downing Street have expressed similar views before. This chapter does not intend to give a detailed critique of the entire report but rather zoom into and critique the health sections. The following sets the tone of the ideas that underpinned the report. On page 27 it stated,

*"The more recent instances where ethnic minority communities have rightly felt let down – such as the Grenfell tragedy[17] or the Windrush scandal – sparked genuine national grief over the traumatic loss of lives, and widespread anger and remorse over the mistreatment of fellow citizens. Likewise, the disproportionate impact of COVID-19 on some ethnic minority groups is partly explained by the prevalence of ethnic minorities who work on the frontline and provide unpaid care in multi-generational households. It went on **Outcomes such as these do not come about by design, and are certainly not deliberately targeted.** But, when they do occur, every step needs to be taken to ensure that the reasons why they happened are understood fully, and the causes then acted on to ensure that they are not repeated".*

These statements are not supported by available evidence. There is robust evidence that BAME people have historically been discriminated in the allocation of housing. The Scarman Report in 1981(chapter 4) has discussed this and there has not been much improvement since. There are frequent references to people still living in multigenerational and poor-quality housing. These impacted on their health especially when COVID19 was rampant. Seventy-two victims died in the Grenfell tragedy represented 85 per cent of BAME ethnicity. These people have undergone the application process, vetted, and the tenancy requirement had to be satisfied to be granted accommodation. The building did not come about by some strange accident. Planners, architects and other contractors had to be involved. Not least the dreaded cladding was selected, purchased and installed by the property owners. All these were organised by powerful people

---

[17] At around 01:00 am on 14 June 2017, fire broke out in the kitchen of a fourth floor flat at the 23-storey tower block in North Kensington, West London. Within minutes, the fire had raced up the exterior of the building and then spread to all four sides. By 03:00 am, most of the upper floors were well alight. The fire which destroyed Grenfell Tower in June 2017 was one of the UK's worst modern disasters.

in institutions. On the specific reference to BAME people the lawyers representing the Grenfell residents urged the Inquiry that racial discrimination should be considered as a factor. Munroe and Maragh (2022) (3) made a powerful and moving oral closing submission to the Grenfell Tower Inquiry. The barristers argued,

"people have tried to move around the elephant, under the elephant, squeeze past the elephant; but he very much is still there and is not going away. Racism and discrimination, we say, played a very real part in the response to this tragedy. The playing field was not level. It never has been."

This statement made implicit reference to the manifestation of institutional racism. They added the 'Grenfell Community Impact Assessment' was produced by Kensington and Chelsea police four days after the fire. The Grenfell Inquiry's final report was published in September 2024; it concluded that there were decades of failings by central government and corporations. The Windrush scandal was planned by the Conservative government. This was discussed in chapter 4, some key points are summarised here. Olusoga (2016) (4) related that when the Windrush ship was on its way to Britain the then Prime Minister discussed the possibility of redirecting the ship to East Africa. This indicated the extent to which black Caribbean people were not wanted in Britain. The plan did not materialise and the passengers arrived at Tilbury docks. Gentleman (2018) (5) added that the Home Office destroyed thousands of landing cards. They were records of passengers' names and arrival dates in the UK. The other wider political objective in 2017 was the government's intention to reduce immigration to the tens of thousands. Changes were made with the 2014/16 Immigration Acts and some black British Caribbean people suddenly found themselves labelled as "illegal immigrants". The immigration changes introduced many new checks. It required, among others, employers, bankers, solicitors and landlords, to check if they were dealing with citizens who were legally in Britain. They were required to provide proof of citizenship. In many cases they had to produce passports. These institutions became the eyes and ears of the state and quasi border guards. The end result was many had their bank accounts frozen, lost their employment, housing, and among others difficulties accessing NHS treatment. Some had treatment withheld. Both the Grenfell fire and the Windrush scandal had and are still having a significant impact on BAME people. According to CRED, institutions had nothing to do with the formation of and implementation of these policies. The Commission decided to look the other way and argued that these were not by design and certainly not deliberately targeted. It is incredulous that any group of people with any professional background could arrive at this conclusion in spite of robust evidence to the contrary. Both these events had and still have life changing and disastrous impact on the lives of many.

More controversy followed in the Section on Medicine, NHS recruitment, retention and NHS staff experiences. CRED noted that ethnic minority groups are strongly represented at various grades in the NHS. In relation to NHS pay, recruitment and retention, the report argued that both male and female Asian medics receive slightly higher pay than their white counterparts, with black staff the worst of the three. They do concede that this may be due to the seniority of these Asian medics. Data was retrieved from only a few sources and limited to 2019, but this did not stop the Commission in suggesting that *"such a picture is not consistent with a pattern one might expect of systemic discrimination"*. It goes further and claims the NHS as a *success story* but with negative experiences and difficult career progression, being harassed and bullied more than their white counterparts. In effect CRED contradicts itself. It is not possible for the NHS to be a success story if BAME staff have difficult career progression and are being bullied and harassed. There was much evidence of these during the time COVID-19 was rampant. Moreover, racial harassment is well alive in the NHS and has been for decades. CRED does not discuss the implications of those who have been harassed or the inability or unwillingness of the NHS to eliminate this. In addition, the duty of care of institutions and managers are not discussed. Furthermore, the historical perspective of allocation of BAME staff being directed to the Cinderella and hard to recruit to services has not been taken into context. Hugman (1991) (6) indicated that echoes of colonialism are reproduced in health and care work, indicating the ideology of white superiority was well-established before and is replicated in the NHS. Furthermore, the aim of the welfare state (which led to the creation of the NHS) was to sustain and promote values about family life, national unity and British culture. This meant the values and norms which centred on being white (Williams 1987) (7). The latest available data in 2021 suggested that in about two hundred and fifteen NHS trusts in England there are about eight chief executive officers who are of BAME ethnicity. In 2023, NHS 75 reported that BAME staff remain proportionally under-represented in senior positions (NHS 75. 2023)(8).

CRED was roundly criticised at several levels. Iqbal (2021) (9) made a broader point. She posited that officials at Downing Street have been accused of rewriting much of its controversial report into racial and ethnic disparities, despite appointing an independent commission to conduct an 'honest' investigation into inequality in the UK. Others who contributed stated,

"We did not read Tony [Sewell's] foreword," they claimed. "We did not deny institutional racism or play that down as the final document did. The idea that this report was all our own work is full of holes".

A spokesperson for the race commission however, said:

"We reject these allegations. They are deliberately seeking to divert attention from the recommendations made in the report".

Walker (2021) (10) explained that (CRED) had cited Marmot's study of 2010 but did not consider the 2020 update or a subsequent study he led on structural factors behind varying COVID-19 outcomes. Marmot also criticised the report's contention that health inequalities should be considered an outcome of factors such as deprivation and poor housing rather than ethnicity. Such social conditions

"are themselves the result of longstanding inequalities and structural racism".

CRED, Demir (2021) (11) suggested in terms of accuracy and scholarship, the report failed to draw conclusions based on facts and evidence. The conclusions as many colleagues noted, contradicted much peer-reviewed research carried out by UK academics spanning the fields of health, education, race, sociology, criminology, and others for decades. It also goes against the government's own research like the Lammy Report and UN report of 2019 which condemned entrenched racial discrimination and inequality in the UK. The CRED report is also intellectually incoherent. It denies that structural racism exists in the UK but then recommends what the police as an institution should do to tackle racism amongst its ranks and training. Institutions and organisations in the UK, like schools, universities, the police, the judicial system, the Home Office, the health system and others, can produce negative outcomes for racial minorities. Yet it seems that those institutions cannot be accused of structural and institutional racism. I argue that CRED took a very microscopic view and assumed that institutional racism could be identified in numbers. More fundamentally it not only took a narrow view but more significantly lacked socio-historical and political context. As a BAME male who has worked and survived vile racism in the NHS, according to CRED, I did not try hard enough, should be quiet, take all the abuse quietly, take more initiative and not to worry about racism direct or otherwise. I get sick due to my lifestyle, do not speak English, somehow live in mutigenerational housing, have diabetes, and in the final analysis I made myself poor and then unwell. This is not a reflection of me and my endeavours. Direct and institutional racism blocked me at every stage of my career in the health service and the Higher Education sector. This is not a figment of my imagination or my perception. I lived and survived it. CRED was written to "change the narrative" about racism. It claimed that white people are being "left behind" and provided ammunition for the far-right politicians to use its findings, especially as it was put together by a group of BAME people. The report did not highlight the fact that white people do not experience any form of institutional racism or are "othered". Another suggestion repeatedly made by CRED was the need for more research. This sounded remarkably like the PHE and the Quarterly reports discussed in previous chapter. The timing of both these must be viewed with extreme suspicion. They were both being discussed around 2020 and it seemed very likely the CRED members were influencing the PHE and other health work streams. Now it seemed that every aspect of BAME lives would be placed under the microscope by various academics. No doubt many would be enthused and happy to engage in research not only to generate funds for their departments but also obtain academic credibility for their institutions and themselves. It's clear who will set the parameters and decide where and how this research will be conducted. As Hammersley (1995) (12) pointed out, research has always been a political activity although it pretended to be otherwise. Research is another way of exercising and/or abusing power. Those in positions of power decide what needs to be researched, how, when, where, and by whom. Ahmad (1993) (13) stated research problems do not exist in a vacuum. They are shaped within particular social, economic, professional, political, theoretical, ideological and the historical context. The identification of research issues is like the construction of social problems. In relation to race and health, Ahmad continued, research has become a major industry. Its benefits to BAME people in terms of understanding illness or improving health care are minimal. It usually benefits the powerful institutions and often to keep status quo or reinforce existing stereotypes.

COVID-19 and the CRED report

As COVID-19 arrived in January 2020, it saw Britain in the grip of fourteen years of austerity. It has eroded social and economic development as an epidemic of funding cuts resulted in a precarious public sector labour market. Household and disposable income were significantly reduced and resulted in an explosion in the use of food banks. The Guardian estimated in 2021 alone that 50,000 deaths are linked to austerity. Children services have moved to crisis intervention and the government was blamed for stripping away services for vulnerable families. Different regions of the country suffered more, with areas in the north of Britain being disproportionately impacted. Some commentators suggested that cuts have destroyed the fabric of society as we know it. All these have impacted on all the social determinants of health and health care provision. Shortfall in social care funding impacted and is still impacting on NHS services. This has led to increased demand for NHS community services, increased emergency and unplanned care admissions. There is also a serious matter of delayed discharges due to a shortfall in social care support. A strong body of evidence indicates that BAME people suffered much more from the austerity programme. This was compounded by the hostile environment, Windrush scandal, and the rise in anti-immigrant hostility during the run up to and after the European Referendum. There was an increase in hate crime and general intolerance of BAME people. In 2020 we were to be hit by COVID-19 virus (see chapter 8). In chapter 7 the state of Britain's readiness was discussed. It concluded

"The UK's preparedness and response, in terms of its plans, policies and capability, was currently not sufficient to cope with the extreme demands of a severe pandemic that would have a nationwide impact across all sectors".

This was followed by another warning in May 2018. Professor Sridhar, a prominent leader in global public health at Edinburgh University, predicted with uncanny accuracy how the next major threat to UK health would evolve. These warning signs were completely ignored. More was to follow in the months preceding the weeks and months before the virus entered British shores. The then Prime Minister wanted to carry on as normal and believed that Britain will not be severely impacted by the virus. National borders were left open and sports activities continued as normal. Data from GOV.UK 17 November 2023 indicated that 233,791 people died from COVID-19. This is the highest in Western Europe.

This context was irrelevant to the CRED report. In the cursory discussion on COVID-19 (another odd decision as Britain was in the grip of the worst pandemic for decades if not centuries), it summarised the extent to which BAME people were affected during the first and second waves. The causes (like the PHE reports), it argued, were the risk of infection, geographical factors, such as living in a densely populated inner-city areas, socio-economic characteristics, and living in larger and multigenerational households. It remarked that death rates of various BAME sections of the population being infected and dying from COVID-

19 has changed from wave 1 to wave 2. During the second wave Bangladeshi, Pakistani, and Indian men and women were over-represented in mortality figures. There were significant variations between the other BAME and white people. It does not explain as to how such a drastic change has occurred during such a relatively short timescale (wave 1 and wave 2), other than it was driven by the risk of infection. CRED repeated the same findings from the previous PHE and the Quarterly reports. The four Quarterly reports were published in October 2020, February 2021, September 2021 and December 2021. The purpose was to outline cross government work that were being taken to address the disparities highlighted by the PHE reports. The PHE, Quarterly reports, and the publication of the CRED were absolutely determined to take racism and all its manifestation out of the equation. Although the CRED report was published March 2021, its core messages seem to have reverberated around the Department of Health and its entourage. It cannot be ruled out that the ideas of the CRED found their way in the workings of the PHE reports of June and August 2020 and other reports. It cannot be a coincidence that statements like "this is opposite that has been known in previous years..." and *experimental, selected and estimated national data* were used to underplay the real impact of direct and institutional racism in the wider social institutions and the NHS. The other common denominator during the COVID-19 and the release of the CRED report in March 2021 was the then Prime Minister Boris Johnson. He wanted to "change the narrative" on racism.

Decades long and credible research were set aside, and other research were called for to understand *further* the cause of these disparities. The latter is another method of kicking racism in the long grass and designed to delay action to address the wider social determinants of health. The focus was to medicalise the entire situation to promote vaccine confidence and uptake in BAME communities. In essence the overwhelming message was to underplay the socio-economic and other determinants of health and maximise the benefits of the vaccine. Racism as a major causation of ill health by Ratcliff and the 'weathering' defined as the psychological effects of living in communities that bear the brunt of racial, ethnic, religious and class discrimination as identified by Geronimus is not considered. CRED supported the zooming in local communities and

"Improve reach, understanding and positive health behaviours".

Over and above the promotion of the vaccine there was much more emphasis on the individual themselves. Some of these strategies ended up blaming BAME people for not leading *positive health behaviours* and other situations that led to them being infected by the virus. Many sections of the Asian community have lived in larger multigenerational households for decades and have linguistic needs that do not chime well with information that were distributed. A significant number of Asian people work in local shops, taxis, are bus drivers and occupations that bring them in very close contact with the public. This increased the likelihood of being infected. This section of the population having suffered disproportionately by over a decade long austerity measures, and the voluntary sectors which were rooted in the local communities have been stripped of funding by the local authority. The initiative of having *community champions* were simply a short-term knee jerk response and too late for many who have succumbed to the virus. There was a distinct impression that BAME people must fit the health system rather than the other way round.

There are other serious shortcomings in the COVID-19 section of the CRED report. There is no reference to the high number of BAME staff who were infected and died in the course of their duty. This has been discussed (see chapter 10), nor the fact that many BAME staff were disproportionately allocated to 'red' wards (with patients who were seriously sick with the virus) with poorly fitting or inadequate PPE. Risk assessment was seen by many as a paper exercise. Bullying, frequently reported in the NHS, is referred in general terms and relied on evidence from the NHSE. This information was received from NHS organisations on a self-assessment basis. So, the possibility of an under-reporting due to fear of recriminations cannot be ruled out. For many BAME staff racist bullying has been a recurring problem for decades. These are only marginally highlighted in the CRED report. It portrayed the NHS as a success story with significant over-representation of ethnic minorities in high status professional roles. This is significant. Ethnic minorities are in clinical roles and are significantly under-represented in management roles. This was frequently referenced by most BAME clinicians who felt their views were not reflected by management. Furthermore, the historical and contemporary evidence do not support that. A health circular in 1977 indicated that BAME staff were under-represented in senior management roles. In an open letter to the then Chief Executive of the NHSE the Chair and Chief Executive of Ethnic Minority Network (2021) (14) pointed out that in March 2021 there are 231 NHS Trusts and Foundation Trusts in the NHS in England and only eight are of BAME ethnicity.

The difficulties in purchasing, distributing and allocating of PPE do not feature in the report. CRED report continued its absurdity. Over and above CRED getting the diagnosis and treatment wrong, on page 15, four key recommendations are proposed. They are to build trust, promote fairness, create agency and achieve genuine inclusivity. Trust, a five-letter word, has very deep meaning and has been the subject of much discussion for centuries. Trust is associated with words like reliability, truth, strength, confidence, honesty, mutual respect, warmth, and amongst others not to cause harm. Trust takes years to develop and must be earned. It is easy to lose trust and almost impossible to regain it. Events over decades if not centuries, have not provided an environment within which trust will develop and grow between many BAME people with British institutions and its citizens. How do ideas of white superiority and the reliance of pseudoscience to prop up the view of inferiority, the enslavement and the systematic attack on BAME people chime with building trust? How does the segregation of Black and Asian soldiers during both world wars and the overt discrimination in all aspects of life after the wars promote trust? How does the constant and disproportionate stop and search of particularly Black and Asian people fit in the promotion of trust? During the COVID-19 lockdown era, most crime was at its lowest, yet BAME people were still disproportionately stopped and searched. How does the rise in hate crime during the run up to and after the European Referendum and the Windrush Scandal which resulted in criminalising black British people build trust? Does the way NHS staff being systematically discriminated and bullied to look after patients with poor and/or ill-fitting PPE build trust?

CRED, NHSE and BAME staff not a "success story"

NHSE's (2023) (15) analysis showed more than two fifths (42 per cent) of doctors, dentists, and consultants, and almost a third (29.2 per cent) of nurses, midwives, and health visitors are of BAME ethnicity. The figures showed an increase in representation at board level – including executive board roles, but BAME staff remained under-represented in senior management positions. The number of Black and minority ethnic board members across all NHS trusts have increased to 13.2 per cent in 2022, up from 12.6 per cent the year before, and almost double what it was in 2017 (7 per cent). Many of the board roles are made up of non-executive directors and are occupied by BAME people. The number of BAME very senior managers has increased from 9.2 per cent to 10.3 per cent (an increase of 51 – up from 290 in 2021 to 341 in

2022). Baker (2022) (16) explains this phenomenon. In the early 2010s there was a rise in the proportion of staff that were of EU nationality. After the EU referendum the proportion had fallen slightly. The proportion of NHS staff reporting as Asian nationality has risen from 4.0 per cent in 2016 to 8.6 per cent in June 2023. Reported African nationality has risen from 1.8 per cent to 3.8 per cent since 2016. Reported EU nationality rose from 2.9 per cent in 2009 to a high of 5.6 per cent in 2017. Since then, it has gradually fallen and was 5.2 per cent in June 2023. Campbell (2022) (17) concurs indicating that more than half of all doctors joining the medical register last year qualified outside UK and European Economic area.

This is not a new phenomenon. At the very inception of the NHS, medical schools underestimated the number of medical staff that was required to meet the needs of the NHS (see chapter 2). The shortfall was rectified by recruiting mainly but not exclusively doctors from the Indian subcontinent and parts of Africa. Nurses were recruited from Mauritius, Sri Lanka, West Indies, and some other colonies. Most doctors and nurses were directed towards the Cinderella services. During the COVID-19 era many were in front line roles and in the sharp end of treating patients. Many were provided with ill-fitting and unsuitable PPE. Rimmer (2017) (18) commented on a report from the House of Lords. It concluded there is long-term sustainability of the NHS, highlighted concern at the absence of any comprehensive, national long-term NHS workforce strategy. Much of the work being carried out to reshape the workforce is fragmented across different bodies with little strategic direction from the Department of Health. Little appears to have changed BMA's media team in (2022) (19) and noted chronic staffing shortages is still underpinned by a lack of effective workforce planning by Government. On 30/6/2023 Prime Minister Sunak announced a fifteen-year plan to train and keep more NHS staff. More doctors and nurses will be trained as well as new roles will be created to work alongside them.

Clews (2021) (20) posited in relation to nurse recruitment have been active in 'red' countries. This meant these are the countries that are in greater need of their own staff. However, Britain is actively recruiting from Nigeria, Ghana, and Nepal. They are the largest number of overseas staff joining the Nursing and Midwifery Council (NMC) register between April 2021 and March 2022. Gulland et al (2022) (21) added another method of facilitating overseas recruitment. To supercharge the recruitment drive they allege that the entry criteria for nurses from India and the Philippines have been "weakened".

There are other reasons for the increasing reliance on overseas nurses. In 2016 the government stopped the bursary system for nurses and a few other disciplines. The bursary of about £8000 was critical in recruiting nurses and its withdrawal resulted in a 40 per cent drop in applicants. This measure was very short-sighted and did not consider that student nurses must attend clinical placements to develop their skills. They need to travel at different times due the shift system. This resulted in a significant shortfall of trained nurses some years later. The main reason for the cancellation of the bursary was due to the austerity measures. The bursary was partly reintroduced in February 2019 with nurses all receiving £5,000 but specialist students like mental health receiving the additional £3,000. This received a lukewarm response. Britain's exit from the European Union resulted in many EU staff exiting the NHS that resulted in a drastic shortfall in staffing. This led to a sharp rise in overseas recruitment. This is much quicker and cheaper. It saves the taxpayer billions as they have not paid for the primary, secondary, and further training of these professionals. There is an uncanny similarity here with the very early days of the NHS in 1948. Soon after its inception many staff were unhappy with the working conditions and pay. They were getting organised and were demanding better conditions of service. In its objective to keep cost down, the government embarked on a programme of recruiting overseas staff. Ireland was the first port of call, but this was inadequate to fulfil the demand. This is very similar to the events (in 2023) of strikes by nurses, medical staff, and other allied professionals looking for better pay and working conditions. More nurses, doctors, and other allied staff are now being recruited to rectify the shortfall. NHS hierarchy has learnt many decades ago that it is a very quick fix and there is no need for any long-term workforce planning. As per its modus operandi it is much more convenient and cheaper to launch recruitment drives from overseas. Some would argue that the pandemic made NHS staffing shortages worse. King's Fund in 2015 and RCN in 2011 revealed that these staffing shortages pre-dated the pandemic. The combination of austerity measures and Britain coming out of European Union placed the NHS and the social care sector in unprecedented pressure. Ashworth (2023) (22) argued "austerity had battered the NHS even before the coronavirus".

Once overseas staff are recruited, the next question is how they are treated, and why many often leave prematurely. In relation to BAME staff the first alarm was raised in 1977 after the publication of the Race Relations Act 1976. It stated that BAME staffs were under-represented in senior positions (this has not changed in 2013) and this is not due to lack of qualification or experience. A series of initiatives have been launched since then. Most were short-lived and were not proportionate to the problems BAME staff were and still facing. There have been many high-profile cases of various NHS trusts being taken to employment tribunals and found to have treated staff unfairly due to their race. This is only the tip of the iceberg. Many cases do not reach the tribunal, and others may well be resolved internally and with the completion of a non-disclosure agreement. This keeps recurring and it seems that not much learning is taking place, and the perpetrators face little or no sanction. Fast forward January 2023, White and Thomas (2023) (23) from The Independent found a third of BAME staff have suffered racism, bullying as the NHS fails to address *systemic levels of discrimination*. This has not improved in the last five years with 30 per cent saying they have been targeted in the last year compared to 20 per cent of white staff. As discussed in the last chapter this was exacerbated during the pandemic and resulted in a disproportionate death of staff of BAME ethnicity. NHSE argued that the BAME workforce has increased but Campbell (2022) (24) reported that 25 of non-executive directors have seen discrimination at work or experienced it themselves. NHSE (2023) (25) supported the above. The latest workforce data on February 2023 indicated that there was an increase of BAME staff in the NHS and conceded that is likely due to an increase in international recruitment. Ethnic minority staff who believe their employer offers equal opportunities for promotion or progression to all staff has marginally increased but remains lower than in 2018. Reports of abuse, bullying and harassment from patients, their families and the public have increased for all staff since 2021. The number of staff reporting discrimination by a manager or another member of staff has also increased for all since 2020. NHSE reported an increase of white staff in bands grade 6,7,8,9 but a decrease of BAME staff in bands 6,7,8,9 (the higher the number the higher the status). It is noteworthy that very senior managers have the highest number of 'unknown' ethnicities in both clinical and non-clinical roles. This has been consistent in the NHS for decades. In 2023 the NHSE defined very senior managers (VSMs) as "someone *who holds an executive position on the board of and NHS trust or NHS foundation trust or someone who although, not a board member, holds a senior position typically reporting directly to the chief executive. The chief office, finance officer, chief nurse, and similar senior staff employed by the CCGS are also VSMs*".

More worryingly, women from a black background and from an Arabic background, experienced high levels of discrimination from managers or team leaders but for many BAME and ex-NHS staff it simply confirmed what I have known for at least four decades. The other aspect is the frequency of abuse and discrimination by staff, patients, families and members of the public is not unexpected. This is due to the overt hostile environment promoted by the government and well assisted by sections of the media. The increased harassment in the wider society towards East Asians and other minority ethnic people were reproduced in the NHS. Patients and NHS staff are influenced by these hostilities, and they take this to work and/or to receive health care. The NHS is a microcosm of the wider society, and its values are reflected in the NHS. The systematic racism faced by staff and patients have been well discussed. The NHSE commented that despite increased board diversity, the gap between whole workforce and board members diversity is widening. The largest gap is at the executive level. The majority of the BAME board members were non-executive directors (NEDS). They are part-time with less power and authority in the overall functions of the board. The contribution by NEDS, Kark and Russell (2018) (26) observed, were variable in holding the executive team to account. Where they were confident and tenacious, there was greater depth and discussion of all issues, including on clinical matters. Limited knowledge of patient safety among Board members, especially NEDs, restricted their ability to ask challenging questions about safety issues. After observing many board meetings, this chimes with my view and I also noted the chasm between the discussions at the Board meeting and the realities on the cold face of care delivery. The NHSE stated its commitment to promote in this case race equality in the NHS. The latter is loosely governed and funded by the Department of Health and Social Care. They decide the goals to be achieved. Hospital trusts are independent organisations and run by the board under the leadership of the chief executive. They decide how goals are reached. This means that the DHSC has very limited power or authority to compel trusts to make equality improvements (Kark and Russell). All that is left is the power of 'working together' 'collaboration' and use 'examples of good practice'. There is no evidence that these strategies have resulted in any sustained improvements.

CRED on mental health services

The CRED report made some much unsubstantiated claims on mental health services. It claimed on page 200,

"There is no overwhelming evidence of racism in the treatment and diagnosis of mental health conditions".

This conclusion was drawn after the commission *heard evidence*. It is not clear if evidence was received after interviewing BAME service users, carers, staff or psychiatrists who have considerable expertise on this field. Although this has been an ongoing concern, caused angst and trauma for many, CRED does not provide any alternative explanation. In 1973, I started training to become a mental health nurse. The hospital was an 800-bedded psychiatric institution in the outskirts of Glasgow. Almost all the patients there were white working-class men and women. They were detained under various sections of the Mental Health Act. This meant they were in hospital against their wishes. Male and female patients were locked up in separate wards and any contact with a different sex was strictly forbidden. Once admitted they stayed there for months, if not years. This was replicated in many similar institutions across the country. The prevailing view was that white working-class people have low pay and low skilled jobs, not very educated, have too many children, more likely to commit crimes and have a propensity to become mentally ill. Some men were admitted due to engaging in anti-social behaviour and some women for having children out of wedlock. The treatment was to lock them away and medicate them. Most if not all these institutions were located out in the countryside, out of sight and out of mind. There was outrage by some academics and activists, but the practice continued for decades.

Unbeknown to me at that time, I was witnessing what Geronimus called "weathering". This meant the psychological effects of living in communities that endure the most of, in this case, was institutional social class discrimination. Many Irish people, particularly men, were seen as aggressive, not intelligent, alien, and inferior. Many were referred to as "Paddies" and not by their names. They received more medication and were subject to informal segregation. After the Second World War many people from parts of Europe, especially Polish men, were over-represented in mental asylums. The last few decades saw BAME patients (especially young black men) being over-represented in mental health hospitals across the country. There is evidence in Western Europe and United States that Black and minority patients are over-represented in the coercive end of the mental health system.

Thomas and Sillen (1993) (27) provided a historical perspective. During the days of slavery, white supremacists used pseudoscience to support that black people cannot manage freedom and are likely to become mentally ill. They went further and developed a term 'drapetomania'. This was a diagnosis used to label black slaves when they ran way or escaped from slavery. The treatment was to re-capture them and keep them as slaves. Some of these ideas have been and are reflected in Britain. BAME men especially experience high rates of detention under various mental health legislation, have a diagnosis of severe mental disorder, and receive more physical treatments like medication. They are more likely to be restrained and sent to medium or secure units. Detailed research has been available since the 1980s by various specialists like Fernando, Littlewood and Lipsedge, Bhui, Sashi Sachidharan, and many others. They all postulated that institutional racism was and is a central cause of the over-representation of BAME people in mental health services. In 2003 a subsidiary of the Department of Health published *Inside Outside* that provided a comprehensive account of racism within mental health services. It argued that institutional racism was a central cause for the over-representation of BAME within mental health services. The other key publication was the Blofeld Inquiry (2003) (28) also called the David Bennett inquiry. This was launched after a black male patient died while being restrained by nurses at a hospital. One of its recommendations was that all staff in mental health services should be trained to tackle overt and covert racism and institutional racism. GOV.UK (2022) (29) posited the detention rates for Black African-Caribbeans were almost five times, and Black Africans highest, than white people. Chinese and some Asian people are the lowest. Detention rates for all ethnic groups are likely to be underestimated because not all NHS providers submitted complete data during the period covered. Evidence of discrimination during detention is hardly likely to be seen on the detention papers. Practitioners are unlikely to write on these legal papers when white working-class men and women were detained at disproportionate numbers in huge psychiatric institutions.

"He/she is a working-class people, who are dangerous to themselves and to others",

Or in the 1970s and 1990s and continuing,

"He is big black and aggressive therefore we will need to detain and sedate him as soon as possible".

Crude stereotypes that are prevalent in the wider society have seeped into the wool of psychiatric practice and have become an integral part of the assessment and treatment process. Racist stereotypes are seen as facts. These alongside the involvement of the police provide a toxic environment in which assessments are conducted. Furthermore, it is well known that social-economic factors caused by institutional racism have had and are still impacting on all determinants of ill-health. The other fundamental problem is in the very knowledge base of what constitutes mental illness. This is heavily based on Eurocentric values. These have roots in colonialism and still prevalent in a much covert way. I have on many instances heard of consultant referring to *"cultural issues"* about BAME patients. When asked what this means statements like *"low intelligence"* *"culture shock"* and *"odd life style and/or drug taking"* are made. These labels were not and are not applied to white working patients. Thus, the prevalence of racist stereotypes, adverse socio-economic conditions and the Eurocentric values which underpin psychiatric practice contribute to the repeated and persistent over-representation of BAME people within the mental health system. I have repeatedly heard nursing and medical staff making stereotypical comments about BAME patients and prescribe tranquilising medication even when the patient (s) are not *"uncooperative or difficult"*. This can also occur with the most junior staff like nursing assistants with words such as,

"I don't like the look of him, he needs to be in a side-room, in case he starts playing up".

Every aspect of the person's behaviour is observed within the context of being *"unpredictable"* or *"aggressive"*. Had the CRED commissioners met with a group of BAME people who have been in mental health hospitals, they would have most certainly come to a different conclusion. Another GOV.UK Rapid Review (2023) (30) prompted by a series of patients' safety in mental health inpatient settings, but little reference was made about BAME patients experiences. The report does not make any reference to the David Bennett Report (2003), Count me in Census (2005-2010) or the Inside/Outside reports (2003). Racism within mental health services have been ignored again.

Maternity services

Roxby (2023) (32) discussed the report called for faster progress to tackle *appalling* higher death rates for black women and those from poorer areas in childbirth. According to the Women and Equalities Committee, racism played a key role in creating health disparities. Many complex causes are *still not understood,* and more funding and maternity staff is also needed. The report refers to data from 2018-2020 and revealed that black women are nearly four times more likely than white women to die within six weeks of giving birth, with Asian women being 1.8 times. Women from poorest areas of the country, where a higher proportion of babies belonging to ethnic minorities are born, are two and a half times more likely to die than those from the richest. BAME women made the following comments,

"I felt they stereotyped me", "they weren't really kind or caring- they ignored my pain and they dismissed me when I cried and begged for pain relief. They actually didn't believe I was in pain."

The system was *"working against me"*. My pain was *"actively dismissed"*. There are stereotypes of black women not feeling pain, and being quite aggressive and loud, very strong, so we are able to take more pain. Black and Asian women are dying from the same causes as other women but more frequently. The most common include heart problems, blood clots, sepsis and suicide. CRED would argue that their report was concluded in March 2021. The disproportionate number of BAME women dying within weeks of giving birth has been going on for at least twenty years. Parsons et al (1993) (33) pointed out "the view of many health professionals is that there is nothing wrong with the services provided. It is those people with 'special diets', 'strange religious practices' or 'funny maternity habits' who have the problem". There are still elements of these today in many aspects of care delivery, from mental health, COVID-19, elderly care, and haemoglobinopathies. In maternal care, over the last twenty years, many women have been critical of the maternity care. The problem encountered by black and ethnic women must therefore be set in this wider context, rather than being seen as a minority issue. Maternity care needs of ethnic minority women are often based on stereotypes rather than on reliable information. This statement was made in 1993. Unfortunately, judging by the experiences of women in the latest report, little seems to have changed. Mundasad (2023) (34) reported from NHS Race and Health Observatory, it raised significant concerns about a focus on skin colour in routine health checks for newborns. The Apgar score[18] is determined by a series of quick assessment immediately after birth. The assessment is based traditionally, includes checking if the baby is "pink all over". The report questions its relevance and accuracy or some babies belonging to ethnic minorities. It also concluded that most healthcare professionals said it was harder to identify jaundice in babies belonging to ethnic minorities. There are calls for better training for staff and making use of handheld meters to measure jaundice levels. There are also the wider issues that have been discussed in chapter 3, i.e. the Kirkup and Ockenden reviews.

---

[18] It describes the condition of the newborn infant immediately after birth and when properly applied is a tool for standardised assessment. Score between 7-10 is deemed to be normal. The scores are based on heart rate, breathing, muscle tone, reflex responses and skin colour. All carry 2 points.

NHSE is investing £165 million in the maternity workforce and was promoting careers in midwifery with an extra 3,650 training places. On a very basic level, how much money and/or training do staff member need to accept that when women say they are in pain or need help; they must be taken very seriously? It can be argued that NHSE is simply sticking plasters in a system that has had problems for decades. Fourteen years and counting of austerity have left an indelible mark on the state of the NHS and on the social determinants of health. Funding and more trained midwives may be of limited value if expectant mothers are living in poverty, deprivation, poor or overcrowded housing, and among others living in polluted areas. Maternity services have been failing BAME women for decades and this cannot be due to actions or lack of actions by a few isolated individuals. These are long-standing and institutional failures by all sectors from education, housing, welfare, access to information, sensitivity of services provided and expectant mothers being at the very centre of the process.

In all the above service provision inequalities, there were and still is very clear evidence that entrenched stereotypes and Eurocentric ideologies about BAME groups featured significantly in the way staff responded to patient's needs and requests. These false views had detrimental implications for the 'care' patients received. On the much wider level, the latest publication by Finney et al (2023) (35) in the latest publication EVENS puts the final nail in the CRED's coffin. It provided the most up-to-date and comprehensive evidence of ethnic inequalities in Britain. It is timely and highly pertinent to contemporary social and political debates on ethnicity and racism after the pandemic. This provides a template of how research should be conducted with BAME people. It was the largest and most comprehensive survey to document the lives of ethnic and religious minorities in Britain during COVID-19. This unique research employed cutting–edge survey methods to ensure a robust data set. It collaborated with thirteen leading voluntary, community and social enterprises. The sample 14,200 participants of whom 9,700 identified as members of ethnic and religious minority groups and allowed comparison in experiences. Data was collected by a questionnaire which was developed in collaboration with local BAME organisations. This was complimented by Computer Assisted Telephone Interviewing and was offered in 14 different languages. In some cases data was collected by face-to-face interviews. The target group was widened to include those who identified themselves as Jewish, the white British group and any other white background, any other mixed or multiple background, and any other ethnic group. The age groups ranged 18 to over 64 included women and across several parts of Britain. Data was collected between March and November 2021. The key findings are summarised. These findings should not come to any surprise for any BAME person who is acutely alert to the contemporary situation. Racism is alive and well; many have experience discrimination before and during the pandemic. Many experienced physical assaults as well as the wider ramifications in education, employment, poor housing, and of being over-policed and under-protected. BAME people face poorer physical health generally and were adversely impacted by bereavement from COVID-19. There is a view that as regards to some mental health issues minority groups fared better. This can be challenged, as for Hindus there is not a term for depression. The way the person would describe their symptoms is markedly different. There is a growing sense of community especially during times of crisis. Long-standing inequalities continued during the pandemic but these were not exacerbated during that time. However, the persistent ethnic inequalities in socio-economic circumstances have been exacerbated by the pandemic. Despite experiences and many adversities BAME people reported relatively high levels of political trust, high level of engagement and interest in politics.

Finney et al made frequent references to Jewish, Gypsy, Traveller and Roma people. This group has for decades faced many forms of racism and discrimination. This revelation has got some in the media excited and pointed out that not only BAME people suffer for racism. On page 71 and 72 the chart identified "White Irish", "White Eastern European", "Gypsy/ Traveller", "Roma", and "Jewish". It would be interesting to see as to where the black Irish, black Eastern European and other groups would fare in this debate. Essentially not much has changed since the last comprehensive report of Colin Brown by the Policy Studies Institute Black and White Britain in 1984.

Conclusion

This chapter discussed how the government of the day went all out to change the narrative about the extent to which racism and particularly institutional racism exists in Britain. That was the purpose of the CRED report. This was direct reaction to the anti-racist international movement called Black Lives Matter. The movement emerged as a direct result of the killing of an unarmed black man named George Floyd by a white police officer in Minneapolis, USA. There were much media attention and may have caught many racist deniers off guard. The CRED report itself made a series of not only controversial but inaccurate statements. I refer here to the impact of COVID-19 and the NHS. One of the most shocking statements were that Grenfell fire where seventy-two people lost their lives and the Windrush scandal did not happen by design. It claimed that Grenfell tower built itself, aliens placed flammable cladding and many black and minority ethnic people somehow ended up living in these flats. I am surprised that CRED did not blame their 'dysfunctional' family for living in Grenfell tower. The barristers who represented some of those affected by the fire argued that "Grenfell was inextricably linked with race and the majority who died were people of colour". The Windrush scandal was well thought out, planned and systematically implemented by the then Home Secretary. It was an attempt to show to the populist voters that the government was serious of getting immigration to the tens of thousands. The outcome was that many Black people were suddenly declared illegal. As far as my family is concerned, they left Gujarat for Mauritius to provide cheap labour to produce sugar for Britain by choice. Indentured labouring had nothing to do with it. Was it a bad dream my forebears experienced? As for my wife, her ancestors dropped from the sky, landed in Barbados and planted sugar cane to provide bricks of gold for the slave and plantation owners. According to CRED that was just a figment of our collective imagination.

Another argument is that the NHS is a 'success story'. This is based on superficial and selective information and ignored available data since the inception of the NHS. Data emerged by early April 2020 that BAME NHS doctors were dying disproportionately when they contracted COVID-19 while caring for patients. It has been well-documented that especially BAME staff were allocated to 'red' wards with ill-fitting PPE, were bullied, harassed and risk assessments were not always followed by risk management. The history of BAME doctors' experiences since the inception of the NHS was conveniently ignored. My wife and I have collectively spent over seventy years in the NHS and from different vantage points we have concluded that the NHS has never been or will ever be a success story as far as race equality is concerned. As stated before, not one of my line managers gave me any guidance in relation to career progression or what my aspirations were. My wife was an enrolled nurse until she had the opportunity to 'convert' to a registered nurse level. This was only made possible as there was a national drive for the conversion programme. Even then, many white enrolled nurses were the first to get onto the training. My wife and I both experienced racial abuse from patients, so-called colleagues and senior managers.

Institutional and direct racism was there all the time waiting for us to falter. Somehow, we did not.

There is a common denominator when COVID-19 arrived March 2020 and the instigator and publication of this infamous (CRED) report in March 2021. This was then Prime Minister Boris Johnson who authorised the report. I list here some of his major 'achievements': During the height of Brexit talks in August 2019 Boris Johnson tried to prorogue (suspend) parliament. This was found to be unlawful by the High Court. There were allegations about an American businesswoman being offered preferential treatment, Boris was very reluctant to be interrogated by reporters and there was an almighty fall out with his special adviser. The latter broke lockdown rules, there were questions as to who paid for the upgrade of his flat and was fined over the 'partygate' affair. When COVID-19 was knocking at the door he was asleep at the wheels. Advice from WHO were followed late in the day. He went out of his way to shake hands with everybody, mooted the idea of the herd immunity (people will become resistant to the virus once infected) and failed to look at how other countries were preparing to manage the virus. He also missed some COBRA meetings with EU leaders to discuss PPE and ventilators. He was found by parliamentary colleagues to have deliberately and repeatedly misled Parliament about parties he hosted in Downing Street while the entire country was in lockdown. Boris Johnson resigned after more than fifty members of his cabinet resigned after a series of scandals. The highest death rate from COVID-19 in Europe and the number of deaths of patients who were sent to care homes did not feature as a contributory factor to his resignation. These are just some of his abysmal track records. Given that context, he was unlikely to get the CRED report right. So, I need to ask, what is it about racism and its various manifestations that he found so hard to engage with? The next chapter discusses the concept of racism and provides a critique of institutional racism.

CHAPTER 12
DEFINITIONS OF RACE, RACISM AND MANIFESTATIONS OF RACISM

I have made frequent references throughout previous chapters of racism and institutional racism. This chapter aims to define the term 'race', racism and illustrate the different manifestations of direct and institutional racism. The latter is critically analysed. I also provide contemporary examples of both manifestations, but particularly institutional racism. Rutherford (2020) (1) argued that 'race' is a very poorly defined term, it refers to categorisation of billions of people that primarily refer either to geographical landmarks or a handful of physical characteristics – none more so than skin pigmentation. He continued that the dominance of skin colour as a racial classifier is based on historical pseudoscience primarily invented during the years of European empire building and colonial expansion. The primary characteristics of 'race' according to Rutherford are not representative of overall similarities or differences between people and populations. Ahmad (1993) (2) supported these points and explains that race (in the West) has been used to support colonialism of a socially constructed "other", a supposedly "inferior" people or "nation", i.e. white 'race' is "superior" and non-white "inferior". He argued that 'race' has legitimised exploitation based on the "scientific" and "natural" superiority of some over others. Eberhardt (2019) (3) referred to the work of Morton who believed he could determine the intellectual ability of a race by measuring the skull capacity. He concluded that Native Americans were "slow in acquiring knowledge, restless, revengeful and fond of war". Africans were joyful, flexible and indolent; by contrast Europeans had the biggest brains with the English at the top of the heap. These were and are examples of how those in positions of power used pseudoscience to prop up their views. These old 'scientific' views have been repeatedly challenged. Rutherford indicated that these notions have been contested by new scientists for decades. They systematically disputed these findings. Nonetheless these beliefs still circulate in many circles. Leary (2005) (4) quoted James King's work (in the Biology of Race) who opined,

"Race is a concept of society that insists there is a genetic significance behind human variation in the skin colour that transcends outward appearance. There are no significant genetic variations within the human species to justify the division of 'races'".

Similarly, Goodman in Pollock (2008) (5) said racial categorisations are simply not useful for classifying human genetic diversity. Rutherford also challenged the notion of racial purity. This is ahistorical and pseudoscientific. People have moved and reproduced with great vigour and admixture between different and previously separate populations was and is the norm. Much more importantly difference between populations do not account for differences in academic, intellectual, musical or sporting performances between populations. Scott (1999) (6) quoted Hill's work from 1989, who argued that 'race' has been discredited as an acceptable and meaningful category for a number of reasons. This includes the proposition that no race possesses a discrete package of genetic characteristics. Scott goes on,

"There is more intra than interracial genetic variation, and the genes responsible for features such as skin colour are few and atypical and not responsible for disease or behaviour".

Rutherford argued that 'race' is a social construct but also has a biological basis. The latter determines the colour and texture of hair, skin and eye colour and other physical characteristics like our parents. That is not to say that behaviour, attitude and ability have their roots in biology. These are dependent on the complex interplay between 'nature **and** nurture', race or biology do not represent objective reality but instead are meaningful only because people within the society or group accept, they have meaning. These are developed since an early age by a process of socialisation or societal programming. All societies programme people to behave, think and act in particular ways. A simple example would be girls, as soon as they are born would be allocated a pink label and boy a blue one. These are developed as they grow older and the family and wider societal institutions have modes of behaviour and expectations for the girl or the boy. Social constructions are also prevalent in relation to one's age, occupational groups and of course race. Social constructs are the views, attitudes beliefs and stereotypes people have when they see, as stated by Ahmad, in the West by a person who is not white. Stereotypes, Eberhardt elaborated are "pictures in our heads", impressions that reflect subjective experiences but stand in for objective reality. These are continuously replicated by all social institutions like church, education, customs, laws, media and every aspect of the given society. These are reinforced constantly and over time are absorbed consciously and subliminally. Thus, Rutherford pointed out human beings come packed with prejudices. There is no scientific basis to support any of these attitudes or stereotypes.

Definitions of Racism

Leary defined racism *"As a belief that people differ along biological and genetic lines and that one's group's is superior to another group. This belief is coupled with the power to negatively affect the lives of those perceived to be inferior"*.

Another definition is prejudice and power equals racism (Eddo-Lodge, 2018) (7). Ahmad and Jones (1998) (8) added, racist behaviour and thinking have their roots in slavery and imperialism, the ideology of white superiority over other races and the institutionalisation of such ideology in the working of the state and its agencies. Ethnicity and culture are used as a euphemism for biological differences. Pollock supported the above, racism is any act that even when unwitting, tolerates, accepts or reinforces racially unequal opportunities. It allows racial inequalities in opportunity as if they are normal and acceptable or treats people of different colour as less worthy or less complex than white people. She continued that racism is a complex, multifaceted and constantly changing set of practices and beliefs that have the effects of disadvantaging, disempowering, marginalising and stigmatising entire groups. Racism cannot be understood in isolation from wider economic, social and political inequalities. Bohonos (2020) (9) elaborated that racism is the ordinary, the 'normal' way that a given society does business. It is a common experience of people of 'colour' in the USA, Europe and Britain. It serves the interest of both white people in power materially and the working-class white people psychically, and therefore neither group has much incentive to fight or feel any guilt or remorse about it. Rutherford added that racism is a prejudice concerning ancestral descent that can result in discriminatory action. It is a coupling of prejudice against biological traits that are inalterable, with unfair behaviour predicated on those judgements. There is consensus that racism is a highly organised and well-crafted system of race-based group privilege. It operates at every level of society and held together by a sophisticated ideology of 'race' superiority. To be highly organised, the group must have institutional power that is used to develop policies in every institution. Another view, expressed by Fryer (1991) (10), the primary function of racism is economic and political. This is illustrated by the motive in the trade of slavery and the political system to implement the ideology. The political system of racism poisoned and is still poisoning the lives of BAME people in Britain. Racism is a very well organised system and serves the interest of both those in power and the working class. The combination of these two components makes it very difficult to challenge it. People who believe in or practise racism are called racists.

Kendi (11) suggested that a racist is one who supports a racist policy through their actions or inactions or by expressing a racist view. He adds that racism is a marriage of racist policies or racist ideas that produces and normalises racial inequities. This view can be challenged. A policy may not appear to be racist, but its implementation by people who have already been socialised in white superiority can result in different outcomes for those who are not white. Effectively uncritical policy implementation can result in outcomes that are racist. Policy implementers have the discretion to apply a rigid or liberal interpretation of any given policy. The other serious element is the active evaluation of any policy. If the data reveals that the policy is having a disproportionate and adverse impact on say BAME people, then the policy is racist.

Rutherford noted that racists believe they belong to a specific group, the othering of different groups and the displacement of people. Many worry that that their culture would be weakened, in this case (Western culture) also referred to as "our way of life" and would be altered significantly. They believe their rights would be stripped away and given to somebody else. Racism is manifested in a multiplicity of ways.

Direct racism is now discussed and is followed by institutional racism. The latter is critiqued and discussed in more detailed later.

Direct racism according to ACAS (no date (12) occurs when something obvious and blatant is said or done and people are treated less favourably due to their ethnicity or 'race'. Being treated less favourably means one is treated differently and worse than someone for certain reasons (Citizens Advice no date) (13). ACLRC (14) agreed and stated it can be manifested on an interpersonal level and is embedded by individual's racist assumptions, beliefs or behaviour that is supported and reinforced by systemic racism. ACLRC went on to emphasise that direct or individual racism is not created in a vacuum but emerges from society's foundational beliefs and ways of seeing and doing things. Eberhardt added that people are 'programmed' to see in a particular way, that BAME people are not "one of us" and thus belong to an out-group. Most of this programming is based on stereotypes. These images dictate how individuals interpret what is seen. All this is connected to, and learnt from, broader socio-economic and historical factors. ACLRC argued that direct and individual racism is easier to recognise. In the final analysis, direct racism was (and still) leads to institutional racism. Some examples of direct racism are as follows: A Singapore-Chinese student was attacked while walking down Oxford Street by a group of men who told him "I don't want your coronavirus in my country". He suffered a fractured nose and broken cheek bones. A teenage boy spat in the face of the owner of a Chinese takeaway demanding to know if he had coronavirus. A group of children referring to "they are Chinese you need to put your mask on" (from a Muslim family), a Chinese university lecturer was attacked by a group of men, they were saying things like Chinese virus "get out of the country". A Filipino nurse was racially abused by one of his patients. There was another way both these racist viruses impacted on particularly BAME people. In my early days as a nurse, a male patient took pleasure of calling me and overseas nurses 'black bastards'. The other nurses thought it was funny and did nothing. In fact, they made excuses on his behalf. I was frequently told,

"He is a patient and not well" "You should not let it worry you"

The patient used his power as a white person. The ward staff colluded with and supported him. They were bystanders. Furthermore, the Director of Nurse Education refused to accept that my qualifications were of equal value to the Scottish education. She refused to transfer my training although I had more than the required qualifications to the more internationally known Registered Nurse training. She had the power, authority and discretion to do so. This is a manifestation of institutional racism.

A brief history, definition, critique, and recent manifestations of Institutional racism

The very mention of the term of institutional racism brings alarm, anger, anxiety, denial, outright disbelief, and hostile responses. For some it is "not helpful", it means "different things to different" people, it is "politically charged"; the previous chairman of Equality and Human Rights Commission said in 2009 that the police can no longer be "accused of institutional racism" and others say the evidence is "flimsy". For most BAME people it is a fact of life, something is seen, experienced, experiencing and surviving it. It is an ever-present phenomenon appearing in various guises and affects my life daily. In my young days in sunny Mauritius, I experienced this but did not know what it was. This intangible, invisible 'thing' was omnipresent. It was oppressive, weighed on my shoulders, my mind and engulfed every aspect of my life. The same goes for my parents, siblings, extended families and the neighbours. It was relentless. The feeling of powerlessness was palpable. All or most of the local inhabitants were fighting a battle but the enemy was there yet invisible. How can we fight this? We saw white people in positions of power and authority. Through a series of institutions, they had best jobs in the banks, key positions in government, had white only schools, 'occupied' the best beaches, had big cars, and walked around with an air of absolute arrogance. They commanded respect from all non-white people. I distinctly recalled the interaction between the local inhabitants and the white plantation owners. At the end of the week, groups of workers would gather at a location to pick up their wages. The white man would arrive with his entourage and the workers would be called in turn to collect their hard-earned pay. Almost all the workers on being called would remove their hats and give a bow of respect to the white man. There was no response from the latter. He sat there on his high chair and looked down at these workers. He was the only white man there and he had absolute power and control. The workers would be called; they made their way to the front where the helpers would count and hand over the cash. They would return to sit at various spots and waited for the trucks to take them home. This was a weekly event. Even at the young age of sixteen or seventeen, I had an inkling that there was something very wrong here. These episodes I witnessed several times, and they had a deep impact on me. I could not name it, until decades later. It was a manifestation of institutional racism in a very brutal form. No words were spoken, there was no need to. The workers unquestionably 'knew' their place and the white man certainly knew his. This was normalised. The workers knew that any deviation from this would result in serious consequences of the loss of work, and income and they would not be able to provide for their families. It was traumatic to witness the extent to which in the late 1960s how the ideology of white superiority was so entrenched. It was painful to witness the oppressed respecting the oppressor. Nothing else would have been tolerated by the powers that be. This was an economic form of institutional racism.

There was another way in which institutional racism deeply impacted on me. This was through the education system. College students and I had to endure an extremely Eurocentric curriculum. Power this time was exercised through the education system. We were taught English Language, and literature, French Language and literature, British history and Christian religion. Other subjects were mathematics, geography and chemistry. All except the French were taught in English. These were the subjects that we would be examined either at the School Certificate Level or the Ordinary Level at the end of the year. The papers would be marked in Cambridge in Britain. This was the only avenue available to progress into our lives. If we did not, we would end up working in the sugar cane field as our fathers. Somehow, we all knew that there was no option and the Eurocentric education was the only method available to escape not only poverty but the relentless oppression by the white rulers in Mauritius. Looking back now, I escaped poverty but not racist oppression. As a group of young people, we used to complain about this. An old man may be in his sixty's overheard us and interjected. I am not sure if he was literate or numerate and he said, "if you all want to get out of poverty, you need to stop complaining and get on with it or, you will all end up like me". We were stunned. We all knew that he was right. We were trapped. We did not like it but there was no alternative. The educational institution's objective was to inculcate us into our inferiority and white superiority. Our language, religion, country and history were of no importance. We were told Britain was the centre of the universe and we believed it. We were not offered another perspective. The British Council had libraries, and all the books were about life in Britain, and I recalled reading legal books there as I had early aspirations to become a lawyer. During the early 1960s the political climate began to shift.

Many Mauritians unhappy with the absolute and relentless domination of the minority white people began to demand self-rule. This got stronger and stronger, and it was inevitable that the British would have to concede. The British demanded the leasing of one of the smaller Mauritian islands. The order was blunt, "no lease of the island will result in no independence". They wanted the island to relocate a naval base. The Mauritian negotiators reluctantly agreed. I then saw the last days of British rule.

Mauritius became independent on 12 March 1968. The first few years after independence were awful. Deep recession set in, and unemployment was at a record high. At the same time there were major recruitments events by a few countries. There was Australia (it wanted white people only and excluded most Mauritians) and the others were France and Britain. Large scale recruitment events were held around the country and well-advertised in the media. Most were recruiting nurses for the NHS. Consequently, many young Mauritians left primarily for Britain to train as nurses. The vast majority were directed towards mental health, learning disability, or the elderly care sector. Furthermore, many ended up training for a qualification that was not recognised outside Britain (Enrolled Nurse/ bedside nurse). I was one of them. It cannot be ruled out that the Eurocentric curriculum was designed to fulfil this aim. Mauritians left in droves rescued the NHS in their hour of need and worked in sectors that not many local British people wanted to. Those of us who qualified as registered nurses (in the Cinderella services) would reach the charge nurse level (in charge of a ward) and a very tiny number would reach lower level of senior manager roles. The majority were dumped some decades later through various NHS reorganisations and more specifically the nurse's grading system. Reorganisations, whenever they took place, often impacted adversely on the few low level BAME managers. Many were made redundant. This was recurring theme. The grading system was designed to provide a career structure of nurses and other group of workers. It would reward nurses for the skills rather than their roles. The grades were from A to I. The lowest was A and the highest was the I grade. The higher the skill level the higher the grade. Its implementation led to dissatisfaction from many, especially BAME nurses. It took place in plain sight. All the good intentions, Equal Opportunities Policies and the Race Relations Act of 1976 fell by the wayside. It resulted in most Mauritians and other BAME nurses being denied their appropriate grades. Most were allocated F grades, and some were offered protected pay for a few years. Less experienced and recently qualified nurses were granted the G grades and above; they were mostly white. They ended up managing the very charge nurses who trained them a few years ago. Many overseas and BAME nurses who were not treated fairly left either through early retirement, redundancy, and others left for the private sector. None of these would be in research. This proposal would not see the light of day. I saw all these as they evolved in front of me. These unpleasant episodes were, on reflection, not unexpected. Given that the ideas of white superiority were well entrenched in all aspects of British life and the NHS, the overwhelmingly white managers interpreted the criteria of the grading as they saw fit. They had all the discretion to do and used their authority to delay or dismiss challenges to their decisions. Appellants were given complex forms to complete, and, in many cases, this process took years to resolve. In my case, for once, Lady Luck showed up. I was appointed as a nurse teacher in June 1988. I can draw similarities here with what occurred to my family decades ago. My forbears were duped and transported by the British from Gujarat to Mauritius to toil the sugar cane fields. In the early 1970s, I was duped by the British authorities to come to Britain, in a deep countryside in Ayrshire and provided with a training that was not recognised internationally. Later, I was directed towards mental nurse training. Effectively, I was part of the 'reserve army' as referred to by Doyal and

Pennell (1979) (15) and the view of Hugman (1991) (16) that the echoes of colonialism are reproduced in health and care work. There are very few very senior BAME managers or Chief Executive Officers in the NHS to date.

Some of these experiences resonate with my wife's experience in Barbados. The white people had the pleasure of the best beaches and lived in parallel lives to that of the local people. There were the red-roofed colonial mansions surrounded with lush gardens that were kept in a pristine state by the local people. That was the nearest they would get to the plantation owners. As in Mauritius, sugar was the main product and the local people were employed to cultivate, harvest and load the sugar cane in trucks. Most if not all the local people worked in the cane fields. The ideology of white superiority was well entrenched there too. My wife's entry into the NHS was like mine. She started in a mental hospital in deep Warwickshire as an auxiliary nurse, then enrolled nurse and eventually as a Registered nurse in mental health nursing. For both of us, there is no need to define institutional racism. We saw it, lived it, and still surviving it. This continues throughout the NHS and our lives. The island of Barbados was and is known for the official form of institutional racism.

In 1661 Barbados became the first English colony to pass a comprehensive Slave Code (University of Maryland blog) (17). Dabiri (2021) (18) expanded that before 1661 the idea of 'white people' as a foundational 'truth' did not exist. The Barbados Slave Code officially known as *An Act for Better Ordering and Governing of Negroes*, announced the beginning of a legal system in which race and racism was codified into law, and from where our understanding of 'white' and 'Negro' as separate and distinct races found its earliest expression. Dabiri continued, this went on to inform the Jamaican Slave Code (1684) and on the mainland of what would become the United States of America. The new ideas that were spreading throughout the English colonial world at that time continue to shape the power structure that determined 'black' and 'white' relations to this day. The Slave Code described black people as "pagans, barbaric, uncertain and dangerous kind of people". It was supposed to protect slaves from cruel masters but in practice extensive protection was provided for the slave owners not the slaves (Encyclopaedia, 1992) (19).

As regards to British rule of India, Shilling (2003) (20) quoted from Sinha (1987) the British justified its rule of Bengal through a Victorian gender ideology. Bengali men were seen as effeminate and identified defects in Indian society which made it unfit for self-rule. These men were not fit to share political and administrative power because of their questionable masculinity. Victorian ideology held that early sexual experience was meant to corrupt the moral fibre of men. Bengali men were suspect because of their inability to exercise sexual restraint. This was exhibited by the practice of child marriage. These men's physique was constructed as "puny" and "diminutive" (Visram, 2002) (21).

My experiences in Mauritius and in Britain suggested that institutional racism is less overt, far more subtle, and not easily identifiable in terms of specific individuals committing the acts. Its impact is without doubt very profound. To locate its definition, (Kendi) referred to Carmichael and Hamilton in the 1960s. They differentiated direct and institutional racism.

"When in the city of Alabama a white person firebombs a black church and kills black people, the media reports the event and is followed by disbelief, rage and sadness by those who are not affected by the fire".

This was described as an act of direct racism. However, when many babies die each year because of lack of proper food, shelter, medical facilities and poverty, no one notices and there is no outcry. It is not newsworthy, and the public's reaction is relatively muted. This is how institutional racism operates. It works quietly, continuously, and creeps up on people without them knowing it. By the time the person realises it is very late in the day and very difficult for individuals to challenge the system and the people in the system. The individual has to challenge the institution, and this can be very stressful, expensive, and take a huge toll on the person and their families. It is a collective behaviour, a workplace culture, supported by a structural status quo and a consensus often excused and ignored by authorities (Eddo-Lodge). She used the terms institutional and structural racism interchangeably and argued dozens, hundreds and thousands of people with the same biases joining together to make organisations and act accordingly. Everyone in the organisation is expected to conform to these values and norms or face failure. Policies are also made by usually the same people (Kendi) and all in the institution are bound to follow. The economic, political and physical environments are all made by individuals. The objectives of institutional racism are to stop BAME individuals, groups and societies from reaching their full potential and allow others ample opportunities to progress.

Ratcliff (2020) (22) stated government make institutions, policies and practices that produce unequal societies with unfavourable conditions of life for many ethnic groups and they impact on people differentially. Torkington (1991) (23) explained another modus operandi of institutional racism. Administrative systems are run by people (who have already been socialised in the dominant norms, stereotypes, and values of the given society) and the rapidity or sluggishness with which those systems are adopted is indicative of the attitudes held by the administrators controlling them. They have much discretion to act or not to act, to see or turn a blind eye. The enforcement and interpretation of these rules are left in the hands of these people in positions of power. Rules are applied rigidly, partially, selectively or not at all. In the British context, Macpherson (1999) (24) provided a definition in 1999:

"The collective failure of an organisation to provide an appropriate and professional service to people because of their colour, culture, or ethnic origin. It can be seen or detected in processes, attitudes and behaviour which amount to discrimination through **unwitting** *prejudice, ignorance, thoughtlessness and racist stereotyping which disadvantage minority ethnic people".*

It was seen as a watershed moment in British political, social history and race relations. Although it was focussed on the way the police operated, it had implications and ramifications for all institutions. He made seventy wide-ranging recommendations that would be relevant for all. The definition focused on *processes, attitudes, behaviours and unwitting* prejudice. It did not consider that the attitudes and behaviours have been implanted in peoples' minds for centuries as the fact that they have been socialised in the ideology of white superiority. The term **unwitting** provides a get out of jail card for those who harbour discriminatory views, attitudes and have the ability and/or authority to act. Most institutions like health did not believe that any of Macpherson's recommendations were of relevance and simply ignored them. It was a case of collective resistance on one hand, and a lack of political will from the government to systematically implement its recommendations. The result was that hardly any of the 70 recommendations saw the light of day (Parliament, 2021) (25). This concurred with the view that racism in a very well organised and crafted system and institutional resistance is another method of obstructing any change to systematically confront racism. Consequently, status quo is maintained. Another deficiency of the Macpherson report is it does not address the thorny issue of ideology and did not place it into the historical perspective. The ideology of white superiority developed for centuries and supported by pseudo-scientific racism during the days of colonialism and the socialisation process of citizens were not taken into consideration.

I discuss here recent manifestations of institutional racism. Baroness Casey review published a report in 2023 (26). The latter was commissioned in October 2021 by the former Commissioner of the Metropolitan Police (Met) after a series of high-profile cases against serving Met police officers. After extensive investigation the review concluded the Metropolitan Police service is institutionally racist, misogynistic, and homophobic. As regards to institutional racism, Baroness Casey made frequent reference to the Macpherson Report of 1999. She elaborated that not everyone in the Met is racist, but there are racists and people with racist attitudes within the organisation. Black and ethnic minority officers and staff experience racism at work, and it is routinely ignored, dismissed, or not spoken about. Many do not think it is worth reporting. Racism and racial bias are reinforced within Met systems and the Met under-protects and over-polices Black Londoners.

The Children's Commissioner Dame Rachel de Souza (2023) (27) conducted the first project on strip searching because she was shocked and appalled by what happened to the fifteen- year-old black girl. The Commissioner released never-previously-published data on strip searches conducted under stop and search powers by police forces in England and Wales between 2018 and mid-2022. It concluded there were concerning practices around strip searching of children under stop and search and is not isolated to the Metropolitan Police. There are systemic problems with child protection and safeguarding in relation to strip searches of children, including scrutiny of searches conducted. Black children in England and Wales were up to 6 times more likely to be strip searched when compared to national population figures, while white children were around half as likely to be searched. More disturbing revelations were to follow.

Rawlinson (2023) (28) reported that inspectors from His Majesty's inspectorate of constabulary and fire and rescue services concluded that every fire brigade in England is plagued with bullying, harassment and discrimination complaints. Inspectors went further to point that this was the *"tip of the iceberg"*. Some staff were reluctant to speak up after being told it would be "career suicide" to do so. One London fire brigade was placed in *special measures* after a separate report revealed incidents of misogyny, racism and bullying. In cricket, the case of Azeem Rafiq led the England and Wales Cricket Board (ECB) to publish an update on the implementation of cricket's action plan to tackle racism and promote inclusion and diversity at all levels of the game in 2022. The Rugby Football Union (RFU) survey reveals racism experienced by players 'in every area of elite rugby'. The RFU has pledged to ramp up efforts to tackle discrimination in the game after its own inclusion and diversity survey found that "in every area of elite rugby – men's and women's, national team, clubs and academies – players had experienced some form of racism". In football Black players face discrimination on every level: from members of the public, fans in stadiums, abusive messages on social media, and lack of management and coaching opportunities. Ian Wright, a football pundit, discussed the disparate treatment black players received in the press especially when they fail to score goals. To date there is only two black managers or head coach in the English Premiership.

The Illegal Migration Bill

In March 2023 the Illegal Migration Bill was introduced in Parliament with the aim of stopping people from crossing the Channel in small boats. This has become one of the top targets for the government. The Bill plans to change the law so that people who arrive by crossing in small boats cannot claim for asylum or protection. They will be indefinitely removed from Britain to a third country. Rwanda is one of those countries (IRC 2023) (29). The Bill suffered a series of defeats in the House of Lords (Seddon 2023) (30). The Bill was found by the Court of Appeal to be unlawful. The main reason being that Rwanda had not provided enough safeguards to prove it is a safe third country (Taylor and Quinn, 2023) (31). The government appealed against the ruling to the Supreme Court. Despite several defeats, both in the House of Lords and the Court of Appeal, the Bill was passed by Parliament on 17 July 2023. The next day the UN High Commissioner for Refugees (UNHCR) joined the UN High Commissioner for Human Rights (UNCHR) warned that this Bill is at variance with the UK's obligations under international human rights and refugee law. This they argued would have profound consequences for the people in need of international protection. Both organisations argued that seeking asylum is a human right, enshrined by international law to help protect some of the world's most vulnerable people. Office of the United Nations High Commissioner for Human Rights OHCHR (2023) (32) challenged this Bill "Any deportation policy is in direct breach of the UK's commitments and obligations under international human rights and refugee law if it fails to provide for due process safeguards, individualised risk assessments, asylum procedures and adequate protection measures," the UN experts said. McGee (2023) (33) made another pertinent point. Compare this to people who have applied to come to the UK through legal methods and programmes specifically set up by the government, most notably people fleeing Ukraine and Hong Kong, and the difference is stark. The latest figures show that 270,600

Ukrainians have applied for British visas, with 220,300 issued to date. This is supported by Elliot-Cooper (2023) (34) who argued that the Illegal Bill should be called for what it is: racist. He qualified that the "restrictive effect is intended to, and would, in fact, operate on coloured people almost exclusively". However, the Supreme Court on 15 November 2023 unanimously ruled that the Prime Minister's £140 million deal was unlawful because of deficiencies in the Rwanda's asylum system. They went further to reinforce that the plan would be in breach of European Court of Human Right of which Britain is a signatory. After much debate between the Lords and MPs, on 26 April 2024 King Charles gave assent to the UK's government legislation which will allow asylum seekers to be sent to Rwanda. This will now become law in the UK. It is now on hold as the prime minister had suddenly announced that a general election would take place on 4 July 2024.

In chapter four, I discussed the overview of Race Relations after the Second World War and the overt racism faced by BAME people in all aspects of life i.e. in housing, employment, police harassment, underserved in the NHS, just to name a few. Chapter five discussed how BAME soldiers who fought alongside the Allied Forces during both World Wars were seen as inferior, were segregated into different battalions and paid less than their white counterparts. They were seen as aliens and undesirables after the wars ended. There is the ongoing matter of BAME people being disproportionately stopped and searched by the police and the latest attempt by the government to dismiss the existence of institutional racism. In chapter seven, I have already discussed the experiences of BAME patients in maternity, mental health, elderly care, and haemoglobinopathies. Latterly, the arrival of COVID-19 illustrated the most explicit evidence of the manifestation of institutional racism in the NHS. The question is how does racism impact on our health?

Racism as a major determinant of Health

In chapters one and two, I discussed my lived experiences of both forms of racism in Mauritius. Most of us lived in poverty, were permanently sad, angry, anxious, stressed and these without doubt had deep impact on our day-to-day lives. There was a sense of hopelessness, despair, low self-esteem, mental fog and poverty of thought. The ideology of white superiority was conveyed to us by the Eurocentric curriculum in both primary and secondary schools. Our religions were seen as inferior, and we were taught Christianity. History and English Literature were all about Britain. Eurocentric education continued in Britain in nurse education, higher education, and among others the media. It can be argued that this can be a social class issue and nothing to do with 'race'.

There is often an assumption that all people who are poor and live in deprived, isolated, rundown and polluted areas would suffer from ill health and the impact on BAME people would be the same. I refer here to my own experiences and challenge this. Many white working-class people were racist in Ayrshire. They 'knew' that they were superior to us (we were referred to as coloured boys) and made frequent disparaging comments to us and about us. Further in my career, many benefitted from racism after being promoted to jobs full in the knowledge that they were inexperienced compared to their BAME counterparts. The European Referendum exposed more racism especially from the working-class voters. Many voted for Brexit and gave Boris Johnson an eighty-two-seat majority in the 2019 general election. Ironically, they were seriously impacted by the austerity measures implemented by the current government. These two events and many others were underpinned by a strong stench of populism, jingoism, and nationalism. White working-class people may well be poor, live in polluted areas, have significant ill health, poor and low paid employment but they do not experience being 'othered'. They do not experience 'weathering' (see below) to the same extent as BAME people. They have benefited and will continue to benefit from white privilege.

Bassett (2015) (35) posited that the racial structure of society causes and reinforces racism, which can become a powerful cultural script; it permits differences and deadly treatment administered by police to BAME people, prejudicial actions that limit one's opportunities for a healthy life, and exposure to constant micro-aggression that causes stress. Racism as a cause of health disparities is understudied, yet extremely important. Maté and Maté (2022) (36) elaborated. One of the studies from Dr Blackburn found that factors such as poverty, racism and urban blight can directly impact our genetic and molecular functioning. Another researcher, E. Espel, indicated these changes are not small. A neuroscientist, Candice Lewis, researched what is known as epigenetic. Maté and Maté expanded, epigenetics means "on top of" genes. Epigenetics processes act on chromosomes [19] delivering and translating messages from the environment that "tell" the genes what to do. All this takes place without in any way altering the genes themselves. BBC's Martha Henriques explains epigenetics offers "a way of adapting to changing conditions without inflicting a more permanent shift in our genomes [20]. Genes, Maté and Maté argued answers to their environment, without environmental signals they would not function. Life for us would be impossible if not for the epigenetic mechanism that "turn" genes "on" or "off" in response to signals

---

[19] Chromosomes are found in the nucleus of every cell of our body and are made up of DNA, tightly coiled around proteins. We have 23 pairs of chromosomes altogether, and they can only be easily observed during cell division. (The Jackson Laboratory)

[20] the genome is the entire set of DNA instructions found in a cell. It contains all the information needed for an individual to develop and function. (Genome.gov)

from within and from outside of the body. Epigenetics is part of evolution, but it demands a new look at how evolution works.

They referred to a UK study conducted by Dr Szyf on epigenetics workings of a broad range of genes in blood samples of middle-aged British males. The study subjects had begun life at opposite ends of the wealth-to-poverty spectrum, some poor others rich. Gene expression in those who were born well-off was markedly different from that observed in their counterparts who grew up disadvantaged. Another study "found that experiences of racism and discrimination accounted for more than 50% of the black/white difference in the activity of genes that increase inflammation". Long term and chronic stress has a negative impact on immune cell function and may accelerate the ageing process. Stress therefore ages us. Another researcher concluded "Racism Shortens Lives and Hurts Health of Black people by Promoting Genes That Lead to Inflammation and illness".

All the factors discussed above, Ratcliff argued, leads to elevated blood pressure, elevated euro-endocrine hormones, spread of infections and psychological distress. Poor people are more stressed and more ill than any income groups as a direct result in living where they do. In life the poor person's stress can come from all these sources, having to choose between heating or eating, ability to pay their rent, energy bills, food to feed the family, and other obligations. Chronic stress is conducive to poor health outcomes. Ratcliff's research indicated that the cumulative burden weakens the immune system and causes metabolic, vascular, and hormonal reactions. These can result in diminished coping ability and self-efficiency. Wilkinson and Pickett (2010) (37) agreed and expanded, the idea that the mind affects the body has been known since ancient times. They refer to research which supports the notion that stress increases the risk of ill-health and pleasure, and happiness promote well-being. When we are stressed or depressed or feeling hostile, we are more likely to develop a host of bodily ills, including heart disease, infections and more rapid ageing. The body's steady state is disrupted. Stress invokes a flight or fight coping response. Short-term stress helps to prepare for known and unknown events. When faced with long-term stress and trauma, the body goes into fight-flight responses. This response is protective but when this occurs for weeks or months and years, the stress becomes chronic, and the body's responses become damaging. The consequences are the brain function; this is impaired memory and risk of depression. There is deteriorated immune response, elevated blood pressure and higher risk of cardiovascular disease. The high levels of hormones are released by the adrenal glands which can slow recovery from acute stress. Additionally, there is a high level of infertility and miscarriage. Wilkinson and Pickett continued. Chronic mobilisation of energy in the form of glucose into the bloodstream can lead to weight gain in the wrong places and even to diabetes, chronic constriction of blood vessels and raised levels of blood clotting factors which can lead to hypertension and heart disease. Other complications are digestive problems, and damaged cognitive function sleeping difficulties. Chronic stress wears us down and wears us out.

Malik (2024) (38) added another dimension; the concept of 'weathering'. She refers to the work of Geronimus who argued that it is critical to understanding and eliminating population health inequity. It involves not just the physical and environmental stressors of being marginalised, but the psychosocial ones as well. These are high stress, constant vigilance, a lack of trust that things will be ok. This process Geronimus suggested leads to premature ageing, chronic conditions, and early death. The pandemic seems to have vindicated her thesis. It was not the person's age that made them vulnerable to the virus but the continuous weathering. These are some examples of how I experience weathering. Any time a BAME person commits an offence there is a view that I am implicated in it just because I am a member of BAME ethnicity; I am 'guilty' by association. While I was in the process of purchasing a car, the salesman became very interested on how long I had been in Britain. The introduction of social distancing was not a new phenomenon. I have been practicing this for decades. In any form of queues, I keep well away from the person in front. On frequent occasions a white person and I are walking in the same direction, (although few feet away) leads person to move their handbag in front of them and constantly look from the corner of their eyes if I am still there. Travelling on the bus is great, I usually have a seat to myself. Mostly white people prefer to stand rather sit next to me! I am frequently followed in shops and on exiting I always place my receipt in my pocket. On a social policy level, all institutions from education, media, religion, culture, language, and other agencies, promote and sustain the ideology of 'otherness'. There is a legal requirement for banks, solicitors, employers, estate agent, landlords and others to act as eyes and ears of the state to check if they are dealing with someone who is in Britain legally. They have become quasi border guards, and I do not recall any objections by any of these institutions or the people who implement this policy. The cumulative impact of all these result in constant and permanent weathering. Some would respond and say I am "paranoid or too sensitive". This is a form of active denial. No listening takes place and there is no empathy. Anyone who does not believe me needs to read *Black like Me* by John Howard Griffin. He travelled as a white person to various parts of North America. He returned home, darkened his skin, lived with African Americans and learnt the 'lingo'. He had his hair treated to reflect the 'Afro' style. He then proceeded to visit the same places he did as a white person. He published his book of this traumatic journey.

Tucker (2024) (39) added another dimension. In the latest book by Liverpool, the latter investigated the worse outcome of BAME people from COVID-19. She concluded, like Ratcliff, that racism is really a public health crisis. She continued that across the board from infectious diseases to cardiovascular disease, cancer and mental health conditions that BAME people tend to experience the worse outcomes. Racism is a contributing factor to these disparities. Liverpool stated scientific racism underpins lots of beliefs that doctors hold today. She questioned as to why these are still believed given that most of the biological arguments about race has been discredited and it is a social construct. She related the story of how Serena Williams (the professional tennis player and seven-times Wimbledon winner) nearly died giving birth. Doctors ignored her request for a scan for blood clots – a condition for which she takes medication. The point is if this happens to a rich relatively privileged black woman in a well-resourced hospital is ignored, it does not bode well with everyone else. One argument that I have frequently heard is there are many BAME doctors in the NHS, so why does this happen? The entire training programme of NHS staff is still very Eurocentric, managers and the entire management ethos is still underpinned by white superiority. Furthermore, on the wider context, Sanghera reminded us that racism is very much part of the cultural DNA of this country. Andrews argued that Britain's refusal to face up to racism results in delusions, irrationalities and hallucinations. He describes it as psychosis and the costs are being borne by the children of that racist society. We survive but experience all sorts of physical and mental health disorders.

Conclusion

I started this chapter with the purpose of exploring the definitions of terms I have used many times in the chapters above. The term 'race' is defined and the biological versus social constructs are discussed. There is a consensus that race consists of both constructs. Biologically, I look like one or both of my parents, probably about the same height, colour of eyes, etc, but that is not to say that I am inferior or superior to anybody else. The term racism is defined and how powers that be invented pseudoscience racism to prop up the ideology of white superiority. I provide examples of the manifestations of direct and institutional racism. Direct racism is what someone does or says as they see that person as inferior to themselves. Institutional racism is created by people in position of power, and authorities design the rules and policies that have different and adverse impact on others. I discussed how my parents and I were impacted by both these manifestations while in Mauritius. Critically we did not know what it was until decades later. These manifestations continued while I was in nursing, lecturing, and my daily personal life. I discuss how in 1661 the Barbados Slave Code was designed and implemented by the British. It gave legal authority for slave owners to see black people as "pagans, barbaric, uncertain and dangerous kind of people". This code was later taken to Jamaica, and its principles were applied throughout the colonies. The definitions of institutional racism are critiqued, and later examples of its manifestations are discussed. These are in the police, Fire Service, vulnerable children, sports, and among others the Illegal Migration Bill. It was one of the government's attempts to "stop the boats" and send migrants who arrive by small boats to Rwanda to be processed. The Bill has had much opposition and was deemed to be unlawful by the Supreme Court in November 2023. At this very time Britain took in 220,300 people who were accepted from Ukraine and Russia seemingly without much fuss. In fact, the entire ambiance of the response to the Ukrainian migrant was very different to the treatment meted to others. The resurgence of both forms of racisms is not surprising. It has party politics written all over it. The Conservative party has plummeted in the polls and as it stands the party is unlikely to win the next general election. It is all about votes. This method has well tried and tested before. I list just a few examples. Peter Griffiths in 1964 said "if you want a N****r for a neighbour vote labour". In 1968 Enoch Powell made his 'river of blood speech' and predicted that in years to come the "black man will have the whip hand over the white man". In 1978 the then Prime Minister stated that people are afraid of being "swamped by people from a different culture", and Boris Johnson in 2023 suggested that Muslim women wearing the burkas look like bank robbers and letter boxes. Latterly, the former Home Secretary pointed that the "small boat people has values that are at odds with our country". They all won their seats and occupied very influential jobs in government. Of late those white working-class people who were seriously impacted by over a decade long austerity voted for Brexit and gave Boris Johnson an eighty-two-seat majority in the 2019 general election. These victories were based on a populist, xenophobic and nationalistic agenda. Conveniently forgotten is the impact of COVID-19 on the poorer regions and how especially BAME patients and NHS staff were over-represented in morbidity and mortality. Many were coerced to return to work prematurely (after signs of COVID -19 subsided) and were delegated to 'red' areas. Most feel unable to challenge these practices due to fear of recriminations. Ability or willingness to challenge or complain does not chime well when staff members are reliant on manager's references for renewing their visas, seeking promotion, or alternative employment. Racism experienced by British BAME staff has already been discussed in chapter nine. As of 26 June 2024, in the run up to the general election on 4 July there has been very little discussion BAME death due to COVID-19 and factors associated with it. We have been wiped out of the narrative yet again. Bringing these to the fore does not win votes. By contrast, as per modus operandi there has been extensive debates on immigration. On reflection, I often wonder after experiencing various forms of racism, being 'othered' and 'weathered' for decades how come I did not hit, kick or throw something at somebody. How I managed to do so is a mystery and I cannot explain it. How many other people have felt this or feel that way?

CHAPTER 13
REFLECTION AND CHALLENGES AHEAD

We are nearing the end of our journey, have learnt, thought so much, and now the question is "what do we do?" It is often said, "knowledge without action is useless." This journey started when COVID-19 arrived. As a former nurse, my goal was to document the impact of the virus, with particular attention to its effects on BAME individuals. It soon became obvious that simply presenting the data on its own would be of little use. It needed to be placed in the much wider socio-political, historical and contemporary context. During the exploration of the wider landscape and backdrop, little did I know that major events would emerge and would have significant implications for Britain. On 24th February 2022, Russia invaded Ukraine. The direct ramification was that many Ukrainians were displaced and around 217,000 arrived in Britain. The cost of food rose by 10 per cent and inflation peaked to 5.7 per cent. Both seriously affected the lives of ordinary people and especially those at the bottom rung of the economic ladder. On the 7 of October 2023 Hamas militant stormed into nearby Israel killing around 1200 people and abducting others. These events are still very active and there are fears that one or both could escalate into world-wide conflict.

On the domestic front there was some serious political turbulence. Boris Johnson was the Prime Minister when COVID-19 arrived. He stepped down after a series of scandals on 7 July 2022, but not because of his mismanagement of COVID-19. He also resigned as a Member of Parliament on 9 June 2023. Liz Truss became Prime Minister on 6th September 2022 and was ousted on 20th October 2022. Rishi Sunak was then installed as Prime Minister on 25th October 2022 and pledged to govern with integrity, professionalism and accountability. He set out his five top priorities of which "stop the boats" was one. He became the third prime minister in less than four months. There were other changes at the ministerial level. In health during 2020 we have had five Secretaries of State for Health, some lasting months, and others barely a year. The COVID-19 Inquiry is still in progress, and it seems that some people have lost part or all their WhatsApp messages. Now we have a general election on the 4 July 2024.

As COVID-19 rampaged across Britain, it became very clear that it was having a significant impact on older men, areas in the north, those living in poorer areas, with high levels of deprivation, multigeneration households, and among other factors high levels of pollution. BAME patients and staff were disproportionately represented in morbidity and mortality. This coincided with the Black Lives Matter (BLM) protests. These were sparked by the murder of George Floyd in Minneapolis on 25th May 2020. Both these events propelled a wave of anti-racist protest across Britain. A 'million people march' took place in August 2020. The marchers were people of all ages, ethnicities and genders. These activities gained much media coverage locally, regionally and internationally. The government was caught flat-footed again. Many politicians did not expect this kind of protest and were catapulted into action. There was the usual denial of the existence of any form of racism. The then Prime Minister a well-known racist denier was having none of it. He decided to 'change the narrative'. The Commission on Race and Ethnic Disparities was born in July 2020 during the same time COVID-19 was rampant. The membership of the commission was made up of predominantly people from BAME ethnicities. The report was published on the 31st March 2021 and it was not a surprise the findings indicated that racism exists but institutional racism does not. It claimed the "UK is not deliberately rigged against ethnic minorities". This must have sounded like sweet music to other racist deniers and provided additional support to the right-wingers and the Far-Right groups. To those who experience racism in their daily lives it was a right kick in the guts. The report meant that we as BAME people have got it all wrong. We made it all up.

On reading the report, I felt totally dehumanised. It did not take much time to conclude that the findings were based on very poor evidence and lacked historical context. It stated that the NHS was "a success story" and the Grenfell Tower fire and the Windrush scandal were simply accidents. The ideology which underpinned the report released on 31st March 2021, had its paws all over the data of various PHE and other official reports on COVID-19. The PHE reports were very reluctant to accept that racism is a significant determinant of health and impacted on BAME peoples' life chances. Much reference was made regarding the socio-economic factors, employment, and multigenerational housing, but they failed to highlight the root causes of these inequalities. They were caused by institutionalised racism. As treatment for COVID-19, it consisted of zooming in on BAME communities and to promote the uptake of the vaccine. It was much easier to locate the problem on individuals rather than addressing the oppressive and discriminatory system itself. This has been the modus operandi of most governments for decades if not centuries. Of late all the focus is on sending migrants to Rwanda. Although the Supreme Court has ruled it unlawful as Rwanda is not a safe country. This matter was still being discussed in the House of Lords and the then government was determined to send some migrants there.

Some more political events soon emerged. On 22nd of May 2024, the then Prime Minister Sunak announced a general election. This would be held on 4th of July 2024. As per usual, the issue of migration and "stopping the boats" loomed large during the electoral campaign. One the 5th of July the Labour party won by a majority of 412 MPs. After 14 years of being in opposition the Labour party was back in power with Sir Keir Starmer as Prime Minister. They inherited a country literally on its knees after 14 years of austerity and the deleterious impact of COVID-19. The honeymoon did not last long and over and above having to deal with the aftereffects of the economic and political events both internally and internationally, local elections were held in parts of the country on 1st May 2025. The results shocked the political establishment. The newly formed Reform UK party (previously known as UKIP) won 677 councillors, are in control of ten local councils, have five MPs and two Mayors. On 12th of May 2025 the Prime Minister published a White Paper in immigration. He wanted to "take back control" and stated without rules the country risked becoming "an island of foreigners." He was catapulted into action and specifically pandering to the populist voters. The reaction was swift, and he was accused of using offensive language and imitating the Reform UK policy. The colour of the government has changed but the focus on immigration has not. This is of course not a new phenomenon. Similar actions have been discussed in the previous chapters. Given this complex, hostile and unpredictable ambiance, how can I make a set of proposals or action plans? In the NHS, the Race Relations Act 1976, Race Relations (A) Act 2000 and so many directives and regulations have been ignored and/or resulted in very little improvement.

There are some glimmers of hope that have emerged from unexpected quarters. In 2018, although it has played a leading role in the abolition movement, University of Glasgow (2018) (1) also received significant financial support from people whose wealth, at least in part, was derived from slave trade in the eighteenth and nineteenth centuries. They will discuss how they can engage in reparative justice and other actions the university can take going forward. In a similar vein, Francois (2019) (2) related that Cambridge University has announced that it will finally conduct an "in-depth academic study into ways in which it contributed to, benefitted from or challenging the transatlantic slave trade and other forms of coerced labour during the colonial era". The catalyst of this change was prompted by conversations with students, activists and brave academics. Zacak and Thakkar (3) continued, we are on an ongoing journey to address the legacy of slavery. While we have already taken some actions, there is much more to do, and this is not the end of our work on this important subject. Other British universities have begun to investigate the origins of funds they received and whether they have been generated through historical slavery. Ziady (2020) (4) of CNN Business reported the Bank of England has become the latest British institution to apologise for historic ties to slavery. Several other UK companies acknowledged ties to the slave trade and pledged new financial support to black and minority ethnic communities. Lloyds, one of London's and world oldest insurance companies, and the pub chain Greene King, said they will take steps to make their business more inclusive and provide support for BAME groups. The Church of England has earmarked £100 million pound fund to address its historical links to the slave trade. However, Muvija (2024) (5) reported that this sum is considered too small and needed to be increased to £1 billion pounds.

Actions by individuals is outlined by Owolade (2023) (6). He discussed how Laura Trevelyan a well-known journalist and author discovered that some of her ancestors had owned up to 1,000 slaves on the Caribbean Island of Grenada. Consequently, Laura and six of her family members travelled to apologise for their ancestor's involvement and pledged £100,000 to the island. The Trevelyan family was one of a few individuals, families, institutions, and legislatures that have either considered or fully embraced the policy of reparations. This meant paying money to the descendants of Africans trafficked across the Atlantic Ocean. They were slaves in plantations in the Americas and the Caribbean. The process of reparation according to Trevelyan starts with an apology. The reality is that the Trevelyan's have started the uncomfortable yet important debate. Simpson (2023) (7) points to external pressures being exerted by Caribbean nations. They have decided to bypass the British government and formally demand slavery reparations from Lloyds of London and the Church of England. The Royal family are to be approached as they all have links with the slave trade and the plantation system.

It is frequently said knowledge without action is useless. It would be very easy to conclude that the battle ahead is beyond recovery. This view would be fatalistic and would only benefit the oppressor. As far as individual actions, I enlist some examples of actions that can be implemented by individuals and/or institutions.

DOS
- Read, read, and read widely. Focus on the argument not the writer.

- Exert pressure on politicians by writing letters, lobbying MPs, and seek for the distribution of resources and the taxing of the super-rich. Inequality is no good for anyone.

- Generate activism and mass movement. Draw on convergence of interest. We need to expose discrimination and racism in the wider society and its institutions, including the NHS. Inequality in any form is a failure of morality and humanity. We need to insert these principles in all we do. Inequalities are a drain in resources. All efforts in the NHS need to be focussed on patient delivery not fighting tribunal cases and settling cases with non-disclosure agreements. This is when NHS settles cases by compensating individuals at the taxpayers' expense. Once the cases are 'settled' organisations have no interest in changing the way they work.

- Our struggles are interconnected because we are interconnected. Injustice somewhere is injustice everywhere. Inequalities are like infections, like lies they spread fast. Most are created by people in organisations and are preventable. We need to find some common ground with particularly the working-class people. This can be fraught with difficulties. It was very clear that many voted for Brexit (2016) and for Boris Johnson (2019). However, many turned out for the Black Lives Matter Movement. Sometimes support comes from unlikely sources.

- Institutions must reflect the community we live in. These must be at every level of organisations. This is a means to an end.

- Focus on policy outcome not presentation.

- Only participate in interviewing panels if you have been involved in the entire recruitment process. That is from determining job and personal specifications, advertising, short-listing, interviewing and recruitment.

- Stop individualising issues.

- Revolution needed. All those NHS workers who have retired need to become more active in challenging NHS institutions locally and nationally. We need to ensure out past does not become staff and patients' futures. There is a lot of resources that is not being tapped. Just because some of us have retired on a reasonable pension, racism and any forms of discrimination does not stop. Our future generation will not forgive us for doing nothing. The longer we stay quiet, look the other way and think "I am ok", this does not work for BAME people. It benefits the oppressor. Adapted from Dabiri (2021) and Andrews (2023).

- I am always intrigued as to why men are more interested in their favourite football team, the players they need to buy, or tactics the manager needs to employ. It would be nice to see the same level of enthusiasm to tackle racism and discrimination in any form. We only need a smattering of the same energy and enthusiasm at health institutions events and board meetings! Sports in general, I argue, was an instrument created to keep the working-class people distracted from the real issues that affect our daily lives. We need to move above and beyond that.

- In the NHS a document was released in 1993 entitled *Ethnic Minorities Staff in the NHS. A Programme of Action*. It discussed how goals like recruitment and selection, staff development, racial harassment, appointment to boards, service delivery, doctors, nurses, and management training could be achieved. The programme provides step by step actions to be taken to address the eight goals. The recommendations are as relevant as they were then. It should be implemented.

- Don't assume policies directed at every one will improve the opportunities for those who are most in need.

- There is no evidence that a few modules of Equality Diversity and Inclusion training (via e-learning or few days of 'Diversity training') results in attitude or behaviour change. These are token gestures. It makes the organisations look progressive and is essentially a tick box exercise.

- We must confront racism whenever we find it especially when it is covert or normalised in stereotypes or myths. We must be anti-racist. Seeing BAME faces in high places in institutions might lift our spirits, but if institutions are racist the colour of the person skin is irrelevant. Changing the crew on the ship does not alter the direction of travel. Colonials have always used BAME people to subjugate others who look like them.

- Do not accept that BAME people do not apply for posts. This is a rationalisation for maintaining status quo. Be mindful that 'race' has been discredited as an acceptable and meaningful category. No 'race' possesses a distinct package of genetic characteristics.

- As a BAME person, do not sit on interview panels only at the interview stage. This is management ploy to get them off the hook in the event of the organisation being challenged on their bias or racist recruitment processes.

- Do not fall in the trap that BAME issues should be researched. We are not the problem. Shine the spotlight on how institutions function. Beware research on "ethnicity", it's the wider society and the way its institutions work that need to be researched. Research has always been a political activity although it has pretended not to be.

- Beware those BAME people with a liberal, bourgeois consciousness packed with capitalist ambitions and individualist intuitions. Some merely seek access to the levers of power for themselves.

- Do not assume that staff in the NHS are anti-racists. The NHS is a microcosm of the wider society. Staff and service users come to the NHS with their own values and attitudes. In my lifetime in the NHS, I have seen many policies, good intentions, directives, and even legislation to address racism. Very little has changed. This is due to a distinct lack of sanctions and the powers that be at the national, regional and local levels have simply ignored them.

- Some NHS organisations have an anti-racist statement. Like previous Equal Opportunity and Diversity Inclusion policies, they are just empty statements and a veneer to hide behind.

The struggle for 'race' equality must continue. As Torkington (1991) (8) stated, there are moral, political, economic and social reasons why inequalities should be eliminated in society. Discrimination destroys the moral fibre of society. It is an infective disease whose toxins poison both the oppressor and the oppressed.

On a personal note, my forefathers were in a worst situation. They did not give up. They could not give up. They knew giving up was not an option. Giving up was going backwards. These were their unspoken words. Under the worst possible conditions, they showed resilience that cannot be imagined or quantified. Times are very hard now and may well get even harder. All those who believe in humanity, respect for all, dignity, self-respect, and justice, need to form a coalition and fight for a less unequal world. Whatever small progress we can make will give us momentum. Humanity must prevail. Hope must survive. I may not be around when the promise land arrives, but I hope my children and grandchildren will see the fruits of our labour.

Postscript

I completed the first draft of this book in September 2024. During the publishing process, significant events occurred both in Britain and the United States.

In Britain, a new Labour government assumed office after winning the majority in the general election on 4th July 2024. Sir Keir Starmer became the prime minister. He quickly discovered that he had inherited numerous and significant challenges. Briefly they were the 14 years of austerity which resulted in the rich getting richer and the poor getting poorer. All or most institutions had their budgets cuts by huge margins. The arrival of COVID-19 pandemic found the previous government asleep at the wheels and Britian had the highest death rates in Western Europe. These were interspersed by the manifestation of racism in the police, sports, fire service and among others the NHS. The arrival of people by boats across the English Channel loomed large before, during and continues apace. The new Home Secretary plans to target the business model of the people traffickers and decided to refuse citizenship to those who arrive by small boats. Currently the Prime Minister is embroiled in a row with a most senior judge over a family from war torn Gaza. The judge allowed the family the right to remain after they have applied through the scheme designed for Ukrainians refugees.

In the health care field, there is an ongoing conversation about the ten-year NHS plan, the Assisted Dying Bill is progressing through parliament and the latest rapid review on the state of the NHS has been published. None of these have factored in the needs of people of BAME ethnicity. As a former nurse I note that the Regulator and Professional body for nurses and midwives (NMC) has its fourth chief executive in seven months.

In USA, Donald Trump was elected president for the second time. He has already stated his intention to dismantle diversity programmes and want to trim down the size of his government. This will embolden individuals and organisations in Britain to abandon what limited progress have achieved thus far. On the international stage he plans to impose tariffs on goods imported in the USA.

All these will have profound impact on the fight for social justice across the world. We have been there before and the fight for social justice must continue.

About the author

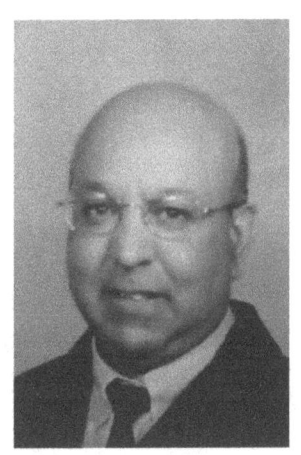

Madhun Foolchand started his NHS career in the NHS in September 1971 in deep rural Scotland. He later trained as a mental health nurse and worked in the Midlands as a charge nurse, nurse tutor and lecturer at a university in the West Midlands. He obtained a Bachelor of Science in Nursing Studies in 1988 and a Master's degree in Educational Studies in 1998. While a lecturer he led several modules in the field of Health and "Race" at various academic levels. He was appointed as a Mental Act Commissioner and visited patients in mental hospitals for over ten years. Other roles before and after his retirement include being an active health campaigner both as a group (Healthwatch) and later as an individual. He has written numerous articles and published his memoir, *Surviving Racism in the NHS*.

Bibliography

Chapter one

(1) Addison, J., Hazareesingh, K. (1984) *A New History of Mauritius*. Revised Edition. London: Macmillan.

(2) Tharoor, S. (2017) *Inglorious Empire. What the British Did to India*. London: Hurst and Company

(3) Doyal, L., Pennell, I. (1979) *The Political Economy of Health*. London: Pluto.

(4) World Book Encyclopaedia (1992) *The island of Barbados*. USA: World Book.

Chapter two

(1) Doyal, L., Pennell, I. (1979) *Political Economy of Health*. London: Pluto.

(2) Ratcliff, K. S. (2020) *The Social Determinants of Health*. Cambridge: Polity.

(3) Sanghera, S. (2021) *Empireland. How Imperialism Has Shaped Modern Britain*. London: Penguin.

(4) Visram, R. (2002) *Asians in Britain 400 Years of History*. London: Pluto.

(5) Snow, S., Jones, E. (2021) *Immigration and the National Health Service: putting history to the forefront. Executive summary 8/3/21* Policy Papers London *History and Policy* Available at:https://www.historyandpolicy.org/policy-papers/papers/immigration-and-the-national-health-service-putting-history-to-the-forefron (Accessed 10 March 2022).

(6) Kushnick, L. (1988) 'Racism, the National Health Service, and the Health of Black people' *Internal Journal of Health Services, Int. J. Health Serv1988*,18 (3):457-70.doi:10.2190/LEUW-X7VW_Q2KD-UML9.

(7) Olusoga, D. (2016) *Black and British. A forgotten History*. London: Pan Macmillan.

(8) Dalrymple, W. (2015) *The Great Divide*. New York: The New Yorker.

(9) Ward, L. (1993) 'Race Equality and employment in the NHS'. In Ahmad, W.I.U. *'Race 'and Health in Contemporary Britain.* Bucks: Open University P 167-182.

(10) Flyn, C. (2018) 'Medics, migration and the NHS'. Part 3 London: Welcome Collection.

(11) "How Asian doctors saved the NHS". BBC News.26/11/2003: London. BBC.

(12) Hiro, D. (1991) *Black British, White British. A history of Race Relations in Britain.* London: Grafton Books.

(13) Department of Health and Social Security (1978) *The Race relations Act 1976. HC (78)36.* London: DHSS.

(14) King's Fund (1990) *The Work of Equal Opportunities Task Force 1986-1990. A final report*. London: King's Fund.

(15) Coker, N. (Ed) (2001) *Racism in Medicine. An agenda for change*. London: King's Fund.

(16) Royal College of Physicians (2020) Survey uncovers years of discrimination against black https://www.rcp.ac.uk/news-and-media/news-and-opinion/rcp-survey-uncovers-years-of-discrimination-against-black-asian-and-minority-ethnic-doctors. 16/10/2020 (Accessed 2 November 2022).

(17) Batty, D. (2020) 'BAME Trainee Doctors in "climate of fear" Over racism'. London: The Guardian 14/2/2020.

(18) Burnet, A., Moorley, C., Grant, J., Kahim, M., Sagoo, R., Rivers, E., Deravin, I. and Derbyshire, P. (2020) 'Dismantling racism in Education: In 2020, The Year of the Nurse an Midwife, "its time"' *Nurse Education Today* Vol 93. Published on-line 2020 Jul 12 doi 10.1016/jnedt2020.104532

(19) DHSS, (1988) New Clinical Grading Structure For Nurses, Midwives and Health Visitors- Implementation Guidance. EL (88) P67 London: DHSS.

(20) O'Dowd, P. (2008) 'Nursing in the 1990's. The introduction of clinical grading caused chaos before Project 2000 revolutionised nurse training'. 12/5/2008. London: Nursing Times.

(21) Daliwal, S. McKay, S. (2017) *The work-life experience of Black nurses in the UK: A report for the Royal College of Nursing*. London: RCN.

(22) NHS Equality Diversity Council (2018) *NHS Workforce Race Equality Standard 2018 Data Analysis Report for NHS Trusts*. London: NHS England

(23) GOV (2023). *NHS staff experiences-Ethnicity facts and figures-* London: GOV.UK. 8/8 2023.

(24) Nursing and Midwifery Council (2022) *Research finds systemic inequalities are driving disparities in regulation*. London: NMC.

(25) Kline, R., Warmington, J. (2024) 'Too hot to handle'. 5/2/2024. *Why Concerns about Racism are not heard or Acted Upon*. Birmingham: brap.

(26) NHS Confederation (2024) 'An invest in Equality, Diversity and Inclusion, urge health leaders' Press Release. London: NHSC

(27) Hugman, R. (1991) *Power in caring profession*. London: MACMILLIAN.

(28) GOV.UK (2022) *NHS workforce: Ethnicity facts and figures (2022)* https://www.ethnicity-facts-figures.service.gov.uk/workforce-and-business/workforce-diversity/nhs-workforce/latest. GOV. UK (Accessed 13 August 2022)

Chapter three
(1) Townsend, P. Davidson, N. (1982) *Inequalities In Health. The Black Report*. London: Penguin.

(2) Department of Health (1992) *On the State of the Public Health for the year 1991. Report of the Chief Medical Officer*. Chapter 3. Health of Black and Ethnic Minorities. London: DOH.

(3) Acheson Report (2005) *Independent Inquiry into Inequalities in Health Report*. London: TSO.

(4) Care Quality Commission (2010) *Count me in 2010.* Nottingham: CQC.

(5) NHS England (2022) *Mental Health Statistics, Annual Figures, 2021-2022.* London: NHSE.

(6) Parliament, House of (2022) *Mental Health Act Reform, Race and Ethnic Inequalities*-Postnote.19th May London House of Parliament.

(7) NHS Race and Health Observatory (2022) *Ethnic Inequalities in Health Care: A Rapid Review Summary.* London: NHS Race and Health Observatory.

(8) National Institute for Mental Health In England (2003) *Inside Outside: Improving Mental Health Services for Black and Minority Communities in England.* London: NIMHE.

(9) National Service User Network (14/12/2021) *Open Letter to Sajid Javid on Institutional racism within Mental Health Act Reform.* London: NSUN.

(10) Fanon Frantz (1991) *Black Skin White Mask.* London: Pluto.

(11) Parsons, L, MacFarlane A, Golding J (1993) (17) In (Ahmad 1993) Ed. *Health and Race in Contemporary Britain.* Bucks: Open University.

(12) Katbamna, S. (2000) *"Race" and Childbirth.* Bucks: Open University.

(13) MBRRACE-UK (2021) *Saving Lives, Improving Mothers' Care. Lay Summary.* Oxford: University of Oxford.

(14) Birthrights (2022) *Systemic Racism, not broken bodies. An Inquiry into racial injustice and Human Rights in UK Maternity Care.* London: Birthrights.

(15) Johnson, W. (2006). 'Watchdog slams maternity unit after 10 women die' *Independent.* 23rd August.

(16) Kirkup, B. (2015) *The Report of the Morecambe Bay investigation.* London: The Stationary Office.

(17) Department of Health and Social Care (2022) *Independent Report: Ockenden Review: Summary of Findings, Conclusions and Essential Actions.* London: DHSC

(18) Blakemore, K., Boneham, M. (1998) *Age, Race and Ethnicity. A comparative approach.* Bucks Open University.

(19) Torkington NPK (1991) *BLACK HEALTH A Political issue.* Catholic Association for Racial Justice London and Institute of Higher Education Liverpool.

(20) Patel, N. (1993) *Healthy Margins: Black elders' care Models, policies and prospects.* In "RACE" AND HEALTH IN CONTEMPORARY BRITAIN. Ahmad WIU. Bucks: Open University

(21) The PSA Research Commission (2019) Black, Asian and Minority Ethnic Older People: How does the crisis in care affect them? Croydon: Advice, Support, Knowledge and Information: ASKI

(22) Lane, C. (2020) *Racial Disparities in drug prescriptions for dementia.* London: University College London.

(23) Anionwu, E. N. (1993) *Sickle cell and thalassaemia: Community experiences and official response* in "RACE" AND HEALTH IN CONTEMPORARY BRITAIN. Ahmad WIU. Bucks Open University.

(24) Public Health England (2018) *Guidance. Understanding haemoglobinopathies.* London: GOV.UK

(25) Parliament House of Commons (2021) *Sickle Cell Treatment*. (Vol 705): Debated on Wednesday 8/12/2021. London: Hansard.

(26) Thomas, T. (2021) NHS staff too slow to treat man who rang 999 from his hospital bed. *The Guardian* 6th April

(27) Hugman, R. (1991) *Power in the caring professions*. London: Macmillan.

Chapter Four

(1) Marshall, T. (2021) *The Power of Geography. Ten maps that reveal the future of our world.* London: Elliott and Thompson Limited

(2) Hiro, D. (1991) *Black British White British.* London: Grafton Books.

(3) Fryer, P. (1991) *Staying Power. The History of Black People in Britain*. London: Pluto

(4) Olusoga, D. (2016) *Black and British. A Forgotten History*. London: Pan Macmillan

(5) The Scarman Report (1981) *The Brixton Disorders 10-12 April 1981*. London: Pelican

(6) Barkham, P. (1999) 'The Stephen Lawrence case Guardian Q and A'. *The Guardian* 23/2/1999.

(7) Barkham, P. (1999) 'Chronology of the Lawrence's' struggle for justice'. *The Guardian* 29/1/1999.

(8) Wikipedia (2024) *Death of Ricky Reel*. Available at: https://en.wikipedia.org/wiki/Death_of_Ricky_Reel. (Accessed 25 August 20240.

(9) Freeman-Powell, S. (2023) '"I still have nightmares" the death of Ricky Reel. Police say they will re-examine the death of student whose body'. Sky News 15/2/2023.

(10) Scraton, P. (2015) 'Policed by Consent?' in White D (Ed) *How corrupt is Britain?* London: Pluto. Page73-84.

(11) Muir, H. (2009) 'In Macpherson's footsteps: A Journey Through British Racism'. *The Guardian* 21/2/2009.

(12) Macpherson Sir William (1999) *The Stephen Lawrence Inquiry-*GOV.UK https://assets.publishing.service.gov.uk/government/uploads/system/uploads/attachment_data/file/277111/4262.pdf Accessed 26/7/2022 (Accessed 9 February 2023).

(13) Parliament, House of (2019) *The Twentieth Anniversary of the Macpherson Report.* 22/2/2019 House of Commons Library. London UK Parliament.

(14) Inquest (2023) *Truth Justice and Accountability. I can't breathe race, death, and British Policing unlocking the truth for 4 years.* Available at: https://www.Inquest.org.uk>police-racism-report (Accessed 12 March 2023).

(15) Gilmore, J., Turfail, W. (2015) 'Justice Denied: Police Accountability and the Killing of Mark Duggan'.in White D (Ed) *How corrupt is Britain?* London: Pluto. P94-102

(16) Dodd, V. (2021) '"Eye Watering": Top Police Officer Laments Rate of Stop and Search on Young Black Men'. *The Guardian* 19/1/2021.

(17) Allen, F. (2014). 'Islam in UK: The role of British Newspapers in shaping attitudes towards Islam and Muslims'. Available at:

https://repository.uwtsd.ac.uk/413/1/Fleur%20Allen%20new.pdf. Accessed 26/7/2022.

(18) History.com Editors, (2010) September11 Attacks London: A/E Television Networks.

History https://www.history.com/topics/21st-century/9-11-attacks Accessed 26/8/2024.

(19) Spalek, B. (2002) 'Hate Crimes Against British Muslims in the aftermath of September 11'. *Centre for Crime and Justice studies*. Number 48. Summer 2002.No 48 Summer 2002.p 20-21 London: Centre for Crime and justice.

(20) Kosh, T. (2017) 'How the 9/11 and 7/7 Terror Attacks have hurt UK Muslims' *Research Gate*. Wales University of Wales. Trinity Saint David. p1-18.

(21) Ray, M. (2024) *London bombing of 2005 Bombing United Kingdom*. London: Britannica.

(22) Hasan, M. (2015) 'Life for British Muslims 7/7-Abuse, Suspicion and Constant Apologies.' *The Guardian* 5/7/2015.

(23) Joint Council for the Welfare of Immigrants (2024) 'Windrush Scandal Explained' London: Web Team JCWI

(24) Gentleman, A. (2020) 'Lambs to the Slaughter' 50 Lives Ruined by the Windrush Scandal. *The Guardian* 19/3/2020.

(25) Merrick, R. (2018) 'Home Office Under Theresa May Destroyed Evidence Able to Spare Windrush Generation From Deportation'. *Independent News* 17/4/2018.

(26) Gentleman, A. (2022) 'Windrush 1:4 Applicants Have Received Compensation'. *The Guardian* 22/6/2022.

(27) GOV.UK, (2023) Home Secretary signal on-going commitment to Windrush generation. London: Home Office. 24/1/2023

(28) Waitzman, E. (2024) *Windrush Scandal and Compensation Scheme.* House of Lords Library. London UK Parliament. 15/2/24.

(29) GOV.UK, (2024) *Home Office in the Media-Windrush Scheme Factsheet.* London: Home office.

(30) Gentleman, A. (2023) 'Unit tasked with reforming Home Office after Windrush scandal being disbanded.' *The Guardian* 19/6/2023

(31) Nagesh, A. (2023) 'Windrush victims being failed by compensation scheme-report'. *BBC News* 17/4/2023.

(32) White, N. (2024) 'More than 50 Windrush victims have died while waiting for compensation governments admits'. *Independent News* 21/1/2024.

(33) Gentleman, A. (2022) 'Windrush scandal caused by "30 years of immigration laws" Report'. *The Guardian.* 29/5/2022.

(34) Matsuda, T. (2021) 'it's time to talk about anti-Asian racism in the UK.' Available at https://www.aljazeera>opinions>its time to talk... (Accessed 10 June 2022).

(35) Ng, K. (2021) 'How British east and south East Asians are fighting racism during the pandemic' *Independent* 13/1/2021

(36) Campbell, L. (2020) 'Chinese in UK report "shocking" level of racism after coronavirus outbreak'. *The Guardian* 9/2/2020.

(37) Morris, J. (2020) (6) '"It's vicious" What it's like living through the UK's coronavirus racism'. *Wikipedia.* 28/7/2020.

(38) Clements, L. (2021) 'Covid in Wales: Racist incidents "take your breath away"' *BBC News*. 9/3/2021.

(39) Wintle, T. (2020) 'Ethnic Chinese is the most common victims of racism in the UK according to a YouGov poll'. *CGTN* 29/6/2020.

(40) Townsend, M., Iqbal, N. (2020) 'Far right using coronavirus as an excuse to attack Asians'. *The Guardian* 29/8/2020.

(41) Parveen, N. (2021) 'Confronting hate against East Asians. A photo essay'. *The Guardian*. 19/5/2021.

Chapter Five
(1) Wilkinson, R., Pickett, K. (2010) *The Spirit Level. Why Equality is Better for Everyone*. London: Penguin.

(2) Visram, R. (2002) *Asian in Britain 400 Years of History.* London: Pluto.

(3) Olusoga, D. (2016) *Black and British. A Forgotten History*. London: Macmillan.

(4) Edencamp (2021) 'Forgotten Friday-Back History during the WW1'. North Yorkshire. Eden Camp Modern History. Blog 22/1/2021.

(5) Williams, C. (2018) *African-American Veterans Hoped their service in WW1 would secure their right at home. It didn't.* Available at: https://www.bunkhistory.org/exhibits/the-lives-of-war-veterans/66/3481 (Accessed 10 March 2020).

(6) Hiro, D. (1991) *Black British, White British. A History of Race Relation in Britain*. London: Grafton.

(7) Fryer, P. (1991) *Staying Power. The History of Black people in Britain*. London: Pluto.

(8) Tharoor, S. (2017) *Inglorious Empire. What the British Did to India.* London: Hurst and Company.

(9) Morton-Jack, (2023) 'Warfare 1914-1918 (India) in 1914-1918 online International' Encyclopaedia of the First WV. Berlin 2023-01-24. DOI: 10.15463/ie/1418.11613. University of Berlin.

(10) Finnigan, C. (2018) '"The story of 1.5 million soldiers that served in WW1 has been forgotten over the years"':Shabrani Basu. London: School of Economics and Political Science.

(11) Sherwood, H. (2018) 'Indians in the trenches: voices of the forgotten army are finally to be heard'. *The Guardian* 27/10 2018.

(12) Parsons, T. (2015) 'Africa's role in WW2 Remembered' Fifteen Eighty Four. *Academic Perspective.* Cambridge: Cambridge University Press.

(13) Buchanan, J. (2020) 'Death Knows No Colour': The Forgotten African Soldiers of WWII' *Global History.* University of Dundee. Scottish Centre of Global History.

(14) BBC. Teach. (no date) *WW2: How did the heroes of the Caribbean help win the war?* https://www.bbc.co.uk/teach/articles/zn96d6f. (Accessed 7 July 2022).

(15) American Air Museum In Britain (No date) '"They treated us Royally" Black Americans in Britain during WW2'. London: Imperial War Museum; London.

(16) Chandra, B. (1989) *India's struggle for independence.* India. Penguin.

(17) Pacific Atrocities Education (2020) 'Forgotten History Pacific Asia War. Episode 32: India's Involvement in World War 2'. San Francisco: Pacific Atrocities Education Podcast.

(18) Fisher, L. (1997) *The life of Mahatma Gandhi*. London: HarperCollins.

(19) Gee, S. (2020) 'Five facts about Indian Contribution During WW Two'.UK: HISTORY HIT

(20) Parliament House of (2021). *Forced Repatriation of Chinese Seamen from Liverpool after the Second World War.* HC (Wednesday 21 July) Volume 699. Hansard: House of Commons.

(21) Grimsditch, L. (2022) 'Striking photos of Chinese sailors living in squalid conditions in Liverpool in a bygone era' *Liverpool. Echo* 17/6/2022.

(22) Blaszczyk, A (no date) The Resettlement Polish refugees after the Second World War. Forced Migration Review. Available at: https://www.fmreview.org/blaszczyk/ (Accessed 11 July 2022).

(23) My Learning, (no date) *The Lasting Effects of World War2-What happened to Poland at the end of the War.* Available at: https://www.mylearning.org/stories/polish-people-in-britain-after-ww2/ (Accessed11 July 2022).

(25) Parliament House of (1947) Polish Resettlement Act 1947 (Pensions). Volume740. Debated on Monday 6/2/1967. Hansard. House of Commons.

Chapter six

(1) Gibbens, S. (2018) 'Britain's Dark-Skinned, Blue-Eyed Ancestor explained'. *National Geographic.* Washington DC.: National geographic.

(2) UCL News (2018) 'Face of Early Brit Revealed'. *University College London.* London UCL.

(3) Rutherford, A. (2020) *How to argue with a Racist.* London: Weidenfeld and Nicholson pub. London.

(4) Fryer, P. (1984) *Staying Power. The History of Black People in Britain.* London: Pluto.

(5) Olusoga, D. (2016) *Black and British. A Forgotten History.* London: Pan Macmillan.

(6) Williams, E. (1944) *Capitalism and Slavery.* London: Penguin.

(7) Doyal, L., Pennell, I. (1979) *The Political Economy of Health.* London: Pluto

(8) Tharoor, S. (2017) *Inglorious Empire. What the British Did to India.* London Hurst and Company.

(9) Sandbrook, D. (2019) 'The Patient Assassin: A True Tale of Massacre, Revenge..' *Sunday Times* 24/3/2019.

(10) Thomas, L. (2020) '7 reasons why Britain Abolished Slavery'.UK: HistoryHit

(11) HistoryHit, (no date). Striking Women / Migration 'Indentured Labourers from South Asia'. UK: University of Leeds, University of Lincoln.

(12) BBC Culture (2020) 'How Britain is Facing up to its Hidden Slavery. History'. London: BBC 5/2/.

(13) Hiro, D. (1991) *Black British, White British. A history of Race Relations in Britain*. London: Grafton.

(14) Mahoney, M. (2020) A 'New System of Slavery'?. The British West Indies and the Origins of Indian Indenture. *National Archives*. London: National Archives. No page Numbers.

(15) Akbar, M.J. (2006). 'The forgotten slaves'. *The Guardian* 12/12/

Chapter seven
(1) Wilkinson, R., Pickett, K. (2010) *The Spirit Level. Why Equality is Better for Everyone*. London; Penguin.

(2) Equality Trust (no date) *UK'S FIVE RICHEST FAMILIES NOW OWN MORE WALTH THE BOTTOM13 MLLIONPEOPLE*. The Equity Trust. Available at: https://equalitytrust.org.uk/news/press-release/uks-five-richest-families-now-own-more-wealth-bottom-13-million-people/#:~:text=Press%20Release

(3) Singh, M. (2024) *'The 2008 Financial Crisis Explained'*. Available at https://www.investopedia.com/articles/economics/09/financial-crisis-review.asp Accessed 29/8/2024.

(4) White, D. (ED) (2015) 'How Corrupt is Britain' in White, D *How Corrupt is Britain*. London. Pluto

(5) The decade the rich won, BBC 2 (25/1/2022) https://www.bbc.co.uk/programmes/m0013xch (Accessed 30 May 2022).

(6) Mueller, B. (2019) What is austerity and how it affects British society? New York: *New York Times* 24/02/2019

(7) Pettinger, T. (2018) 'What is Austerity?' *Economics Help.* Oxford: Oxford University.

(8) Corporate Finance Initiative, (No date) *Austerity. Government Polices that aim to Reduce Public Sector Debt.* (Accessed 25 April 2022).

(9) Elliott, L. and Wintour, P. (2010) Budget 2010, Pain Now, More Pain in Austerity Plan' *The Guardian.* 22/6.

(10) British Association of Social Workers. (2017) 'Position statement on austerity'. Birmingham: BASW

(11) McKee, M., Karanikolos, M., and Stuckler, D. (2012) 'Austerity: A failed experiment on the people of Europe'. *Clinical Medicine* August 12 vol (4) 346-350. doi 10.7861/Climedicine12-4/346.

(12) Casla, K., Burton, J., Donald, A. (2016) 'The UK Government Cannot Reconcile Austerity Measures With Human Rights'. London: *Open Democracy.*20/7.

(13) United Nations, (2008) Fact Sheet No 33. *Economic and social and cultural rights. Frequently Asked Questions on Economic, Social and Cultural Rights.* Geneva Switzerland: UN Office of the High Commissioner for Human Rights.

(14) Hernandez, T. A. (2021) 'An examination of the social outcomes of the 2010 austerity programme in the UK: An analytic narrative approach' .*UK* University of Leicester.

(15) Gregory, A. (2021) 'Austerity in England Linked to More than 50,000 Extra Deaths in 5 Years'. *The Guardian* 14/10.

(16) Parliament, House of Lords (2023) *Mortality rates among men and women: impact of austerity*. 6/1/2023. London: House of Lords Library.

(17) GOV.UK (2022) *The Independent Review of Children's Social Care*. Office of the Children's Commissioner. London: Department of Education.

(18) Economic and Research Council (2018) *Austerity Timeline. Life on the Breadline Coventry University*. London: Economic and Research Council. Available at https://breadlineresearch.coventry.ac.uk/resources/austerity-timeline-2/. (Accessed 18 May 2021.

(19) Toynbee, P., Walker, D. (2020). 'The Lost Decade: the Hidden Story of How Austerity Broke Britain'. *The Guardian* 3/3/

(20) Kingsley, P. (2018) 'British Austerity is Inflicting Unnecessary Misery'. UN Poverty Expert Says'. *New York Times* 16/11.

(21) Oxfam Case Study, (2013) *The true cost of austerity and inequality: UK case study*. Available at: https://www-cdn.oxfam.org>pdf (Accessed 15 May 2021).

(22) Rawlingson, K. (2021) 'Does Income Inequality Cause Health and Social Problems?' London: Joseph Rowntree Foundation.

(23) Runnymede Trust, (2017) *Intersecting Inequalities: The Impact of Austerity on BME Women in the UK*. London Rummymede.

(24) BBC News (2018) 'Austerity and immigration rules concern UN racism official'. 12/5.

(25) Reis, S. (no date) 'The Impact of Austerity on Women in the UK'. London. Women Budget Group. P 1-6

(26) McGuiness, A. (2019) UN Report: Austerity drive has had "tragic social consequences" for UK SKY News 22/5/2019.

(27) Dorling, D. (2023) *How austerity caused the NHS crisis. Open Democracy* .Available at: https://www.opendemocracy.net>nhs-a-and-e-delays-a... (Accessed 5 May 2023).

(28) Whitehead, M., Duncan, W H., Taylor-Robinson, D., and Barr, B. (2021) *Poverty, Health and Covid-19*. Available at: *BMJ* 2021; 372 doi:https://doi.org/10.1136/bmj.n376 (Published 12 February 2021) (Accessed 23 April 2021).

(29) Stuckler, D., Reeves A., Loopstra, R., Karanikolos, M., McKee, M. (2017) 'Austerity and Health: the impact in UK and Europe'. *European Journal of Public Health* Oct 2017 Oct 1.27 supple_4; 18-21.doi:10.1093/eurpub/ckx167.

(30) Marmot, M. (2020) *The Health Gap. The Challenge of an unequal world*. London: Bloomsbury.

(31) Jones, I. (2022) '"Significant' drop in life expectancy in most deprived areas of England.' *AOL News* 25/4.

(32) Independent (2022) Windrush Scandal: Everything you need to know about the... *Independent* Available at: https://www.independent.co.uk>life-style>windrush. (Accessed 16 March 2022).

(33) British Medical Association (2016) 'Health in all policies: health, austerity and welfare reform'. A Briefing From the Board of Sciences. London. BMA Available at: https://www.bma.org.uk>bo (Accessed 2 June 2021).

(34) McLeod, J. (2022) 'Tory austerity "likely caused more death than COVID-19"'. The *National Scotland* 5/10.

(35) IPPR (2020) 'Austerity 'ripped resilience out of the health and care service' before covid-19 crisis hit.' Available at: https://www.ippr.org/media-office/austerity-ripped-resilience-out-of-health-and-care-service-before-covid-19-crisis-hit-says-ippr . (Accessed 10 June 2021).

(36) Finnsdottir, M. S. (2019) *The Cost of Austerity: Labour, Emigration and the Rise of Radical Right Politics in Centre and Eastern Europe*. Frontier Sociology 11/01. Vol 4 Available at: https://doi.org/10.3389/fsoc.2019.00069.

(37) Barrass, S., Shields J. (2017) *Immigration in an Age of Austerity: Morality, the Welfare State and the Shaping of the Ideal Migrant*. Available at: https://doi.org/10.3138/9781487515584-012 (Accessed 13 April 2022).

(38) Simms, A. (2016) 'Austerity, not immigration, to blame for inequality underlying Brexit vote,' *Independent* 8/7.

(39) Hirsch, A. (2018) *BRIT (ish) On Race, Identity and Belonging*. London: Vintage

(40) Mulhall, J. (2021) *Drums In The Distance. Journeys Into The Global Far Right*. London: Icon Books Ltd.

(41) Hayden, S. (2022) *My Forth Time We Drowned. Seeking Refuge on the world's deadliest migration route*. London: 4th ESTATE

(42) Gentleman, A. (2022) 'The racist legislation that led to the Windrush scandal'. *The Guardian* 29/5.

(43) The Joint Council for the Welfare of Immigrants, (2020) *Windrush Scandal explained*.

Available at: https://www.jcwi.org.uk/windrush-scandal-explained Accessed 25/4/2022

(44) Grey, C., Hansen, K. (2021) *Did COVID-19 Lead to an Increase in Hate Crime Towards Chinese People in London?*. Journal of Contemporary Criminal Justice. July 5. Available at: https://discovery.ucl.ac.uk/id/eprint/10134665/ (Accessed 10 August 2022).

Part Two

Chapter eight

(1) Pegg, D. (2020) 'What was the Exercise Cygnus and what did it find?' *The Guardian* 7/5.

(2) ARY News, (2020) 'Professor who predicted corona virus type outbreak slams UK government for "slow" response'. *ARY News* 3/20. .Available at: https://arynews.tv/professor-coronavirus-slams-uk/

(3) Shipman, T. (2020) 'Inside No 10. Everyone is at war'. *The Times* 5/4/2020.

(4) British Medical Journal (2020) 'The UK's public health response to COVID-19. Too little, Too late, Too flawed'. Editorial 15/5.London *BMJ*

(5) Hopkin, J. (2020) 'Brexit thinking poisoned the government's response to COVID-19.' London. London. *School of Economics*.

(6) Taylor, M. (2022) 'The NHS was ill-prepared for Covid-19' London: *NHS Confederation*. 11/1.

(7) Shipman, T. Gregory, A. Leake, J. (2020) 'Stay home alone to save your life, 1.5 million warned' *Sunday Times* 22/3.

(8) Hoernke, K., Djellouli, N., Andrews, L., Lewis-Jackson, S., Mandy, L., Martin, S., Vanderslott, S., Vindola-Pedros, C. (2021) 'Frontline Health Care Workers' Experience with Personal Protective Equipment During the COVID-19 Pandemic in the UK; a Rapid Qualitative Appraisal' .*British Medical Journal.* London BMJ. Open Vol 11(1). Available at: https://bmjopen.bmj.com/content/11/1/e046199 (Accessed 16 December 2022).

(9) National Audit Office (2020) Report. Value for money. The supply of personal protective equipment (PPE) during the COVID-19 pandemic. London. NAO.:

(10) Lee, A. C. K., English, P., Pankhania, B., Morling, J. R. (2020) 11/21. Where England's response to COVID-19 went wrong. National Library of Medicine Online on 11/21.Available at: https://doi.org/10.1016%2Fj.puhe.2020.11.015 (Accessed 15 August 2022).

(11) Oborne, P. (2021) *The Assault on Truth.* London. Simon and Schuster.

(12) Wood, V. (2020) 'Coronavirus: Boris Johnson criticised after "missing five COBRA meetings" at the start of the pandemic'. *Independent* 18/4.

(13) Conn, D. (2020) 'We were packed like sardines: evidence grows of mass event dangers early in the pandemic'. *The Guardian* 3/6.

(14) Tucker, G. Gadher, D., Collingride, J. (2020) 'Flights from Italy, Iran and China still landing.' *Sunday Times* 22/3.

(15) Jit, M., Jombart, T., Nightingale, E., Endo, A., Abbott, S., Edmunds, J. W. (2020). 'Estimating number of cases and spread of coronavirus disease (COVID-19) using critical care admissions. UK February to March 2020.' *Euro surveillance*. Vol 25 issue 18. Sweden

(16) Office of National Statistics (2021) Deaths involving COVID-19, England and Wales Death occurring in March 2020. London: ONS.

(17) Sparrow, A., Campbell, L., Rawlinson, K. (2020) 'UK Coronavirus: Boris Johnson announces strict lockdown across country- as it happened'. *The Guardian*: 23/3.

(18) NHS England (2020) 'Important and Urgent-Next Steps on NHS Response to COVID -19.' 17/3/2020 Leeds. NHS

(19) Smyth, C. (2022) 'Pandemic blamed for increase in death in Heart deaths'. *The Times* 30/12.

Chapter nine
(1) Chaudhry, F. B. Raza, S., Raja, K. Z. and Ahmad, U. (2020) 'COVID 19 and BAME health care staff: Wrong place at the wrong time'. *Journal for Global Health*. Vol 10 P 1-7. USA. International Journal for Global Health. Available at: https://www.jogh.org/documents/issue202002/jogh-10-020358_AU.pdf (Accessed 3 March 2021).

(2) Cook, T., Kursumovic, E., Lennane, S. (2020) 'Exclusive: Death of NHS staff from COVID 19 Analysed.'22/4. London: *Health Service Journal*. Wilmington.

(3) *Is Covid-19 racist?* (2020) Dr Ronx Ikharia.. Channel 4 23/11/2020.

(4) Bhatia, M. (2020) 'COVID-19 and BAME Group in the United Kingdom'. *The International Journal of Community and Social development*. June 25/2020.Vol 2(2) p 269-272 London: Department of Health Policy, London School of Economics and Political Science. London

Available at: http://eprints.lse.ac.uk/106628/1/2516602620937878.pdf (Accessed 23 August 21).

(5) Marsh, S. McIntyre, N. (2020) 'Six out of 10 in UK health workers killed by COVID 19 are BAME'. *The Guardian* 25/5/2020.

(6) British Medical association (2020) 'Remembering the UK doctors who died fighting COVID-19. Memorial Service'. London. News and Opinion.*BMA*.12/4.

(7) Parliament House of Commons (2021) *Frontline-workers-left-risking-lives-to-provide-treatment-and-care*. 10/2/2021. London: House of Commons.

(8) Hoernke, K., Djellouli, N., Andrews, L., Lewis-Jackson, S., Mandy, L., Martin, S., Vanderslott, S., Vindola-Pedros, C. (2021) 'Frontline Health Care Workers' Experience with Personal Protective Equipment During the COVID-19 Pandemic in the UK; a Rapid Qualitative Appraisal'. *British Medical Journal*. London BMJ. Open Vol 11(1). Available at: https://bmjopen.bmj.com/content/11/1/e046199. (Accessed 16 December 2022).

(9) *Why is COVID-19 killing people of colour?* (2021) Harewood, D. BBC1 8/3/2021. London.BBC1.

(10) National Audit Office (2020) *The supply of PPE during Covid-19 pandemic*. HC 961 Session 2019-2021. London: NAO

(11) Parliament House of Commons (2021) Health and Social care and Science and Technology Committee. *Coronavirus: Lesson learnt to date: Sixth Report of Health and Social Care Committee and Third Report of Science and Technology Committee 2021-2022*. HC92.21/9/2021. London: House of Commons.

(12) Pogrund, G., Clover, J. (2022) 'Investigation The PPE Rich List COVID Firms. Unmasked'. London *Sunday Times* 11/12.

(13) Siddle, J., White. C. (2023) 'Exclusive: Tory donor firm paid £11 million to deliver PPE now gets £4.5 million to DESTROY it'. London. *The Mirror*. 14/1.

(14) Oliver, D. (2021) 'Lack of PPE betrays NHS clinical staff'. *British Medical Journal* MJ 2021 372n438. London. BMJ.

(15) Nagpaul, C. (2021) Conference paper at Health and Race Observatory conference 25/5/2021. London

(16) Morgan, E. (2020) 'Discrimination on front line of coronavirus outbreak may be a factor in disproportionate BAME death among NHS staff. 13/5/2020'. London: *ITV News*.

(17) Ramamurthy, A., Bhanbhro, S., Bruce, F., Gumber, A., Fero, K. (2022) *Nursing Narratives: Racism and the Pandemic*. Sheffield Hallam University. Anti-Racism Research Group, Centre of Culture and Media and Society.

(18) Burns, C. (2024) 'Long Covid: Health staff go to court for compensation'. *BBC News*.6/3.

(19) Khunti, K., de Bono, A., Browne, I. et al (2020) 'Risk Reduction Framework for NHS Staff at risk of COVID-19 Infection'p1-10 London: Faculty of Occupational Medicine

(20) Jesuthasan, J., Powell, R.A., Burmester, V., Nicholls, D. (2021) "We weren't checked in on, nobody spoke to us": An exploratory qualitative analysis of two focus groups on the concerns of ethnic minority staff during COVID-19'. London: *British Medical Journal. Open*. 2021; Dec 31:11(12) e053396.11e05396.

(21) ANTIBULLYING ALLIANCE (NO DATE) 'Our definition of bullying'. London: National Children's Bureau.

(22) Arbitration and Conciliation Advisory Service, (2023) 'What bullying is –Bullying at Work'. London *ACAS*.

(23) Elahi, A. S. (2021) 'BAME doctors "still waiting for risk checks"' London: *BBC News* 26/1/2023.

(24) Torkington, N.P.K. (1991) *Black Health. A political Issue*. Catholic Association for Racial Justice. London and Liverpool Institute of Higher Education. Liverpool.

Further Reading
https://www.gov.uk>government>pub>the..The Seven Principles of Public life-gov.uk (Accessed 6 February 2023).

Health Service Executive HSE 13/7/21 COVID-19 Risk Assessment Template. HSE London.

Chapter Ten
(1) Ratcliff, K. S. (2020) The Social Determinants of Health. Looking Upstream. Polity Press. Cambridge.

(2) Northern Health Science Alliance (2021) A year of COVID-19. Regional inequalities in health and economic outcomes. University of Newcastle. UK.

(3) Office of National Statistics (2021) Coronavirus (COVID-19) and the different effects on men and women in the UK March 2020- February 2021. ONS London.

(4) McIntyre, N., Thomas, T., Duncan, P., Swann, G. (2022) What do we know about the 175,000 people who died with COVID-19 in the UK? The Guardian 17/01/2022.

(5) NHSE and NHS Improvement (17/3/2020) Important and Urgent. Next steps on NHS Response To COVID-19. Skipton Leeds.

(6) Spencer, B., Yorke, H. (2022) Hancock Back on Trial. Sunday Times 4/12/2022

(7) HUFFPOST (2022) Government Broke Law By Sending Patients Into Care Homes At Start Of Pandemic 27/4/2022.

(8) Duncan, P. (2021) More care home residents died in the second wave that the first in England and Wales. Guardian 11/5 2021

(9) PHE [1] (2020) Beyond the Data: Understanding the impact of COVID-19 on BAME Communities. PHE. London (June)

(10) PHE [2] (2000) Protecting and improving the nation's health: Disparities in the risk and outcome from COVID-19. PHE London. (August)

(11) Ahmad, W.I.U. (1993) Race and Contemporary Britain. OU Press Bucks

(12) ONS (2022) Updating ethnic contrasts in death involving the coronavirus (COVID-19) England 8/12/2020 to 1/12 2021) ONS London

(13) Nafilyan, V., Islam, N., Mathur, R., Ayoubkhani, D., Banerjee, A., Glickman, M., Humberstone, B., Diamond, I., Khunti, K. (2021) Ethnic differences in COVID-19 mortality during the first two waves of the Coronavirus Pandemic: A national cohort study of 29 million adults in England. European Journal of Epidemiology. 36(6) 615-617.

(14) Scobie, S., Spencer, J., Raleigh, V. (2021) Ethnicity coding in English health service datasets. Nuffield Trust. London

(15) King's Fund (2020) COVID-19 has exposed the 'Stark inequalities' that exist in our society: The King's Fund responds to the PHE report on disparities of the risks and outcomes of COVID-19.

(16) Moore, A. (2020) 2/6/. Exclusive: Government censored BAME COVID-19 review. Health Services Journal. London.

(17) ONS (2021) Ethnic Differences in life expectancy and mortality from selected causes in England and Wales 2011-2014. Experimental analysis of ethnic differences in life expectancy and cause specific mortality in England and Wales based on 2011 census and death registration. July. ONS. London.

(18) ONS (2021) Mortality from leading causes of death by ethnic groups, England and Wales 2012-2019. Experimental analysis of ethnic differences in mortality cause specific mortality in England and Wales on 2011 census and death registration. August. ONS. London.

(19) Sandercock, G., Raghib, A., Mc Conwey, K. (2021) Science Media Centre. Expert Reaction to ONS stats on ethnic differences in life expectancy and morbidity from selected causes in England and Wales 2011-2014. 26/7/2021

(20) Nazroo, J. (2021) Ethnic Inequalities in mortality rates and life expectancy in England and Wales: why we should treat experimental statistics with caution. Published on Race and Health Observatory update on 25/11/2022 London.

(21) ONS (2020) 14/2/2020. Why have Black and South Asian people been the hardest hit by COVID-19. ONS London.

(22) HM Government (October 2020) First Quarterly reports on the progress to address COVID-19 Health inequalities. Race Disparity Unit Cabinet Office. London.

(23) HM Government (February 2021) Second Quarterly reports on the progress to address COVID-19 Health inequalities. Race Disparity Unit Cabinet Office. London.

(24) HM Government (May 2021) Third Quarterly reports on the progress to address COVID-19 Health inequalities. Race Disparity Unit Cabinet Office. London.

(25) HM Government (December 2021) Final Quarterly reports on the progress to address COVID-19 Health inequalities. Race Disparity Unit Cabinet Office. London

(26) Rutherford, A. (2020) How to Argue With a Racist. Weidenfeld & Nicholson. London

(27) Devlin, H. (2021) Gene common in south Asian people doubles risk of Covid death, study finds. The Guardian 4/11/2021.

(28) Scott, P. (1999) in Hood S, Mayall B, Oliver S Ed. Critical Issues in Social Research. Power and Prejudice. OU Press. Bucks

(29) Doyal, L. and Pennell, I. (1979) The Political Economy of Health. Pluto Press London.

Chapter eleven
(1) Commission on Race and Ethnic Disparities: The Report (2021) Race Disparity Unit. 10 Downing Street London.

(2) Turnnidge, S. (2020) Who Is Tony Sewell, the Controversial Head of the Government's New Racial Disparity Commission? HUFFPOST 16/7/2020.

(3) Munroe, A., Maragh, T. (2022) Race and discrimination played a very real part in the response to the tragedy". Grenfell Fire Closing Statement Garden Court Chambers. London.

(4) Olusoga, D. (2016) Black and British. A Forgotten History. Macmillan. London

(5) Gentleman, A. (2018) Home Office destroyed Windrush landing cards, says ex-staffer. The Guardian. 17/4/2018

(6) Hugman, R. (1991) Power in Caring Profession. Macmillan. London

(7) Williams, F. (1987) Racism and the discipline of social policy: a critique of welfare theory. Critical Social Policy 20: 4-29.

(8) NHS 75 England (2023) new figures show workforce is most diverse it has ever been. NHS London

(9) Iqbal, N. (2021) Downing Street Rewrote "independent" Report on race. Experts claim. The Observer News. Guardian. 11/4/2021.

(10) Walker, P. (2021) UK Public Health Expert Criticises No10 race report "Shortcomings" Guardian 7/4/2021

(11) Demir, I. (2021) (17) What is the Race Disparity Unity's Race Report really aimed at? Blog. University of Leeds.

(12) Hammersley, M. (1995) The Politics of Social Research. Sage London

(13) Ahmad, W.I.C Ed. (1993) Race and Contemporary Britain. OU Press. Bucks

(14) https://www.nhsbmenetwork.org.uk/wp-content/uploads/2021/04/sirsimonstevens20210323_820549.pdf

Chairs and Chief Executive Ethnic Minority Network (Accessed 17 April 2023).

(15) https://www.england.nhs.uk/2023/02/new-figures-show-nhs-workforce-most-diverse-it-has-ever- New figures show NHS workforce is most diverse that it has ever been. (Accessed 18 April 2023).

(16) Baker, C. (2023) NHS staff from overseas. Statistics. UK Parliament. House of Commons Library. UK Parliament. London

(17) Campbell, D. (2022) NHS hiring more doctors from outside UK/EEA than inside for the first time. Guardian 8/6/2022.

(18) Rimmer, A. (2017) Poor workforce planning is biggest internal threat to future of NHS parliamentary inquiry finds. https://www.bmj.com/content/357/bmj.j1734 (Accessed 20 June 2023).

(19) BMA (2022) Dependence on international doctors highlights workforce emergency in the NHS, says BMA. https://www.bma.org.uk>BMA mediacentre 5/8/2022. Dependence on international doctors highlights workforce emergency. (Accessed 18 April 2023).

(20) Clews, G. (2021) Concern over numbers of nurses joining UK register from off-limits countries. Nursing Times 19/11/2021

(21) Gulland, A. Wallen, J. Smith, N. Newry, S. (2022) UK "Watered down requirements for overseas nurses in "supercharges recruitment drive. Telegraph Investigation has found, 12/4/2022.

(22) Ashworth, J. (2023) https://www.prospectmagazine.co.uk/opinions/40404/austerity-had-

battered-the-nhs-even-before-coronavirus.-now-we-must- (Accessed 18 April 2023).

(23) White, N., Thomas, R. (2023) NHS Racism shame: 1 in 3 BAME Staff face racism and bullying. The Independent. 24/1/2023

(24) Campbell, D. (2022) 25% of BAME Non-Executive directors have "seen discrimination" at work. Guardian 20/7/2022.

(25) NHSE 75 (2023) NHS Workforce Race Equality Standard (WRES) 2022 data analysis report for the NHS trusts. NHSE London.

(26) Kark, T., Russell, J. (2023) A Review of the fit and Proper Person Test. Commissioned by the Ministry of State for Health. https://assets.publishing.service.gov.uk/government/uploads/system/uploads/attachment_data/file/787955/kark-review-on-the-fit-and-proper-persons-test.pdf (Accessed 29 April 2023).

(27) Thomas, A., Sillen, S. (1993) Racism and Psychiatry. A Citadel Press Group. New York

(28) Independent Inquiry into the death of David Bennett (2003) HSG (94) 27. Norfolk, Suffolk and Cambridgeshire SHA. Cambridge.

(29) GOV.UK (2022) Ethnicity facts and figures. Detention under the Mental Health Act. London.

(30) GOV.UK (2023) Rapid Review into data on mental health inpatient settings. Final report and recommendations. https://psihub.org>other-reports-andenquiries.

(31) Roxby, P. (2023) End racial disparities in maternal deaths- MPS. BBC News 18/4/2023.

(32) Parsons, L., Macfarlane, A., Golding, J. (2023) Pregnancy, birth and maternity services. In Ahmad W I U (ED) "Race" AND HEALTH IN CONTEMPORARY BRITAIN. OU Press Bucks.

(33) Mundasad, S. (2023) Race and Health Observatory "concerns over focus on skin colour in newborn checks." BBC News 12/7/2023

(34) Finney, N., Nazroo, J., Becares, L., Kapadia, D., Shlomo, N. (2023) EVENS. Racism and Ethnic Inequality in a Time of Crisis. Findings from The Evidence For Equality National Survey. Policy Press Bristol University. Bristol. UK

Chapter Twelve

(1) Rutherford, A. (2020) How To Argue With A Racist. Weideneld and Nicholson. London

(2) Ahmad, W.I.U. (ED) (1993) Race and Contemporary Britain. OU Press. Bucks.

(3) Eberhardt, J. (2019) The New Science of Race and Inequality. Biased. Penguin Random House UK.

(4) Leary, J.D. (2005) Post Traumatic Slave Syndrome. Uptone Press. USA

(5) Pollock, M. (2008) Ed Every Day Anti-Racism. Getting Real About Race In School. The New Press London.

(6) Scott, P. (1999) In Critical issues in Social Research. Hood S et al. OU press Bucks.

(7) Eddo-Lodge, R. (2018) Why I'm No Longer Talking To White People About Race. Bloomsbury Press. London.

(8) Ahmad, W.I.U., Jones, L. (1998) Ethnicity, health and health care in Britain in Peterson A and Waddell C (ED) Health Matters. A sociology of Illness, Prevention and Care. Open University Press. Bucks

(9) Bohonos, J.W. (2020) Critical race theory and working-class White men. Exploring race privilege and lower-class work life. https://doi.org10.1111/gwao.12512 (Accessed 24 August 2022).

(10) Fryer, P. (1991) Staying Power. The History of Black People in Britain. Pluto Press. London

(11) Kendi, I. X. (2019) How To Be An Antiracist. THE BODLEY HEAD. Press London.

(12) https://www.acas.org.ukk>race-discrinimation>types-o.. Types of race discrimination at work ACAS. (Accessed 10 February 2019).

(13) Citizens advice.org.uk https://www.citizensadvice.org.uk (Accessed 20 June 2021).

(14) ACLRC aclrc.com forms of racism individual and systemic. https://www.aclrc.com>forms-of-ra... (Accessed 10 June 2021).

(15) Doyal, L. and Pennell, I. (1979) The Political Economy of Health. Pluto Press London.

(16) Hugman, R. (1991) Power in Caring Profession. Macmillan. London

(17) University of Maryland https://blog.umd.edu>slaverylawandpower>barbado... (Accessed 12 January 2024).

(18) Dabiri, E. (2021) WHAT WHITE PEOPLE CAN DO NEXT. From Allyship to Coalition. Penguin Books. UK

(19) https://academic-accelarator.com>Encyclopedia (1992)Barbados Slave Code: Most up to date Encyclopaedia. (Accessed 12 January 2024).

(20) Shilling, C. (2003) The Body and Social Theory. Sage Publication. London

(21) Visram, R. (2002) Asians in Britain. 400 Years of History. Pluto Press. London

(22) Ratcliff, K. S. (2020) THE SOCIAL DETERMINANTS OF HEALTH looking upstream. Polity Press Cambridge.

(23) Torkington, N.P.K. (1991) Black Health: A Political Issue. Catholic Association for Racial Justice and Liverpool Institute of Higher Education.

(24) Macpherson of Cluny, Sir William (1999) The Stephen Lawrence Inquiry. The Stationary Office. London

(25) https://publications.parliament.uk>cmselect>cmhaff: The Macpherson Report 22 years on(2021). (Accessed 13 March 2023).

(26) Baroness Casey of Blackstock Review (2023) Final Report. An independent review into the standards of behaviour and internal culture of the Metropolitan Police Service. London

(27) Dane Rachel De Souza. CHILDREN'S COMMISSIONER (2023) Strip search of children in England and Wales. Analysis by the Children's Commissioner for England. London

(28) Rawlinson, K. (2023) Every fire brigade in England plagued by bullying and harassment claims, report finds. Guardian 30/3/2023

(29) International Rescue Committee (2023) What is the Illegal Migration Bill. IRC. London

(30) Seddon, P. (2023) Migration bill: Government suffers series of defeats in Lords. BBC News 29th June.

(31) Taylor, D., Quinn, B. (2023) Braverman plan to send asylum seekers to Rwanda unlawful Appeal Court Rules. Guardian 29/6/2023

(32) OHCHR (2023) UN expert urge to UK to halt implementation of illegal... https://www.ohchr.org/en/press-releases/2023/07/un-experts-urge-uk-halt-implementation-illegal-immigration- (Accessed 10 April 2024)

(33) McGee L (9/3/2023) The UK pushes a new migrant law slammed as racist, illegal and unworkable. CNN

(34) Adam Elliott-Cooper (2023) Lets call this Illegal Migration Bill for what it is: Racist. The Voice on Line 20/7/2023

(35) Bassettt, M. (2015) 'BlackLivesMatter- A Challenge to the Medical and Public Health Communities' *The New Journal of Medicine/Research and Review.* Vol 372 No12 372:1085-1087DOI: 10.1056/NEJMp1500529

(36) Mate' G., Mate' D. (2022) The Myth of Normal. Trauma, Illness and Healing in a Toxic Culture. Avery. Penguin Random House. USA

(37) Wilkinson, R., Pickett, K. (2010) The Spirit Level. Why Equality is Better for Everyone. Penguin Books London

(38) Malik, N. (2024) Extraordinarily stressed and vigilant? How racism makes people physically ill. The Guardian 4/4/ 20245

(39) Tucker, I. (2024) Extract from Systemic: How Racism Is Making Us ILL. The Guardian 6/6/2024.

Chapter 13

(1) University of Glasgow (2018) University News. University of Glasgow publishers report into historical slavery.

(2) Francois, M. (2019) It's not Cambridge university-all of Britain benefitted from slavery. 7/5/2019 Opinion. The Guardian

(3) Zacak, N., Thakkar, N. https://research.manchester.ac.uk/en/persons/natalie.a.zacek research. add. (Accessed 16 May 2023).

(4) Zaidi, H. (2020) Bank of England joins British companies in apologising for slavery https://www.cnn.com/2020/06/19/business/bank-of-england-slavery-apology/indax.html. (Accessed 16 May 2023).

(5) Muvija, M. (2024) 4th of March Church of England urged to expand fund to address slavery links. Reuters UK.

(6) Owolade, T. (2023) Can money really make amends for slavery? New Review. Sunday Times 2/4/2023

(7) Simpson, C. (2023) Royal family to face demand to pay reparations for the slave trade. The Sunday Telegraph 10/9/2023

(8) Torkington, N.P.K. (1991) Black Health. A political Issue. Catholic Association for Racial Justice and Liverpool Institute of Higher Education. Liverpool.

Further reading
Dabiri, E. (2021) What White People Can Do Next. Penguin Books. Dublin.

Andrews, K. (2023) The Psychosis of Whiteness. Allen Lane Dublin.

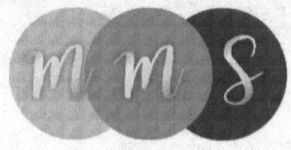

www.marciampublishinghouse.com

www.ingramcontent.com/pod-product-compliance
Lightning Source LLC
Chambersburg PA
CBHW011420070526
44584CB00026BA/3775